What

Love

Looks Like

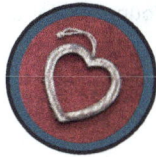

Susie Kinslow Adams

Published in the United States of America

Patches Joyland Press

Susie Kinslow Adams © 2025
Regina Albritton, Editor
Cover and Interior format by C.A. Simonson

Complimentary images from contributing authors
ISBN:978-0-9907700-6-0

Dedication

To the brave souls from near and far, whose shared stories tug at our hearts, assuring us we do not journey alone.

To the faithful friends who have supported this effort with constant prayer and honest feedback.

To Jesus, our Savior, Lord, and Guide. His faithfulness and unchanging love give each story validity and purpose.

Table of Contents

Foreword

I am honored to write a few words about the most recent book of the award-winning author and speaker, Susie Kinslow Adams. I have all her books on my shelf. I was inspired to use many of the truths and concepts I learned from them in my Sunday School class discussions as well as in my Women's Ministry Bible Study. Her books have also benefited me greatly on a personal level.

As you read *What Love Looks Like,* you will find you are peeking into the windows of intimacy where love abides. The many stories are reflections of compassion, endurance, tenderness, mercy, and more. The fruits of the Spirit can be seen growing on the windowsill of the hearts of those who have bravely come forward to share their stories. The sweetness found on every page makes this book truly a worthy read.

Whether you are or will become a caregiver in the future, you owe it to yourself and your family to have your personal information up to date. Susie has offered some valuable helps in the Resource Section at the back of the book. Be assured, I will join the author in praying that God will reveal truth to each reader.

Christian writer and author,

~Donna Barnes

Introduction

My husband, Russell, and I could not have envisioned what God was orchestrating in our lives thirty years ago when he was called to Missouri from California to pastor a rural church. The move meant we would be within two hours' drive time of our children and my mother. Our four children and their families filled the little sanctuary on our first Sunday. Truly, this was the scene movies are made of.

For ten years, short trips home from the coast had offered little time to spend with Mother. They always ended up with her clearly holding back the tears as she waved goodbye. But now that we were close, short trips together, shopping and eating out were all on our agenda.

On Mother's first visit to our home, she became ill and spent several weeks in the hospital. We were not sure at one point if she would come home.

Most of us do not plan to be caregivers. I never wanted that role, especially not to be a caregiver for my mother. She was independent and, from my perspective, had little confidence in my decisions. I never wanted the role, yet I knew a care facility was not an option I would choose.

After several long weeks of ups and downs in the hospital, Mother was released and came to live with us. Physically and mentally for the first few years, she was Mother as I knew her. We finally had time and resources to enjoy trips and daily outings. As her health slowly declined, I automatically took on more of the caregiving responsibilities.

My husband and I were thankful for God's timing in our move back to Missouri. Our story unfolds in *My Mother My Child* as I journal about caring for my mother as she slowly declined mentally as well as physically.

When Mother no longer knew who I was or where she was, I accepted that. Trying to get her to remember something only frustrated both of us. Correcting her was futile, and I knew it.

I wrote this book because I had deep feelings on this subject. I was told my book should be taught to healthcare workers and caregiving families. It never happened so, ten years later, I republished the book providing a discussion guide at the end of each chapter. I'm humbled at the response. Not only did families and individuals find help with caring for the elderly, but my experiences also helped young mothers care for their children.

Through the years, I tried to write a companion guide of sorts to *My Mother My Child*. Something was missing. My titles sounded boring, and my focus was off. In 2024, I received a call from another author, Donna Barnes, asking permission to teach *My Mother My Child*. She had heard of my books through a mutual friend, Jill Maddux. It was clearly God's timing. The prayer support from those two and others was God's call on my heart.

When Donna shared her notes with me, I immediately saw the problem I had been having: LOVE was missing. This was not just a story guide. It should be a tool to use in the toughest of times to remind readers of the truth in Corrie ten Boom's familiar quote: *"There is no pit so deep, that God's love is not deeper still."*

Clearly the Lord's hand directed as stories began to come in – stories of folk who had been or are in the pit with no way out. But God...!

What Love Looks Like is a journey of God's love. His love is the perfect love that grants peace when there is no peace, gives strength when all strength is gone, provides wisdom and clarity as we learn to yield our lives to Him.

Please know that many are praying for you as you soak in His word scattered throughout the stories of those who have been there.

Grief

Grief is not just an emotion
    —it's an unraveling,
      a space where something once lived but is now gone.
It carves through you,
    leaving a hollow ache where love once resided.
In the beginning, it feels unbearable,
    like a wound that will never close.

But over time, the raw edges begin to mend.
The pain softens, but the imprint remains
    —a quiet reminder of what once was.
The truth is, you never truly "move on." You move with it.
The love you had does not disappear; it transforms.
It lingers in the echoes of laughter,
    in the warmth of old memories,
    in the silent moments where
    you still reach for what is no longer there.
And that's okay.

Grief is not a burden to be hidden.
It is not a weakness to be ashamed of.
It is the deepest proof that love existed,
that something beautiful once touched your life.

So let yourself feel it.

Let yourself mourn.

Let yourself remember.

There is no timeline, no "right" way to grieve.

Some days will be heavy, and some will feel lighter.

Some moments will bring unexpected waves of sadness,

while others will fill you with gratitude

for the love you were lucky enough to experience.

Honor your grief, for it is sacred.

It is a testament to the depth of your heart.

And in time, through the pain,

you will find healing

—not because you have forgotten,

but because you have learned how to carry

both love and loss together.

~ Jeff Metcalf

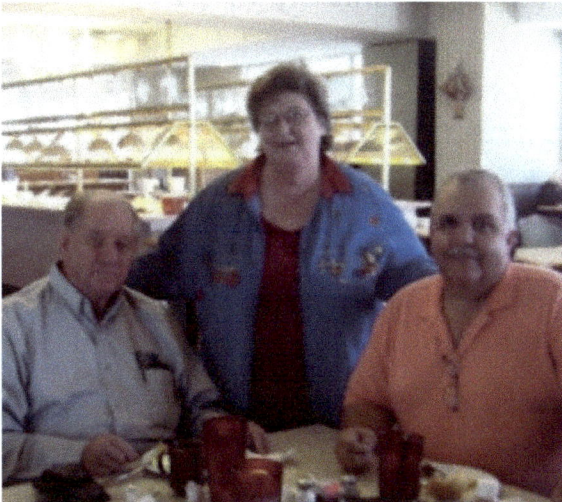

Russell and Susie with Jeff Metcalf

An Encouraging Word

**"For the Spirit God gave us
Does not make us timid,
but gives us power, love,
and self-discipline."**

2 Timothy 1:7 (NIV)

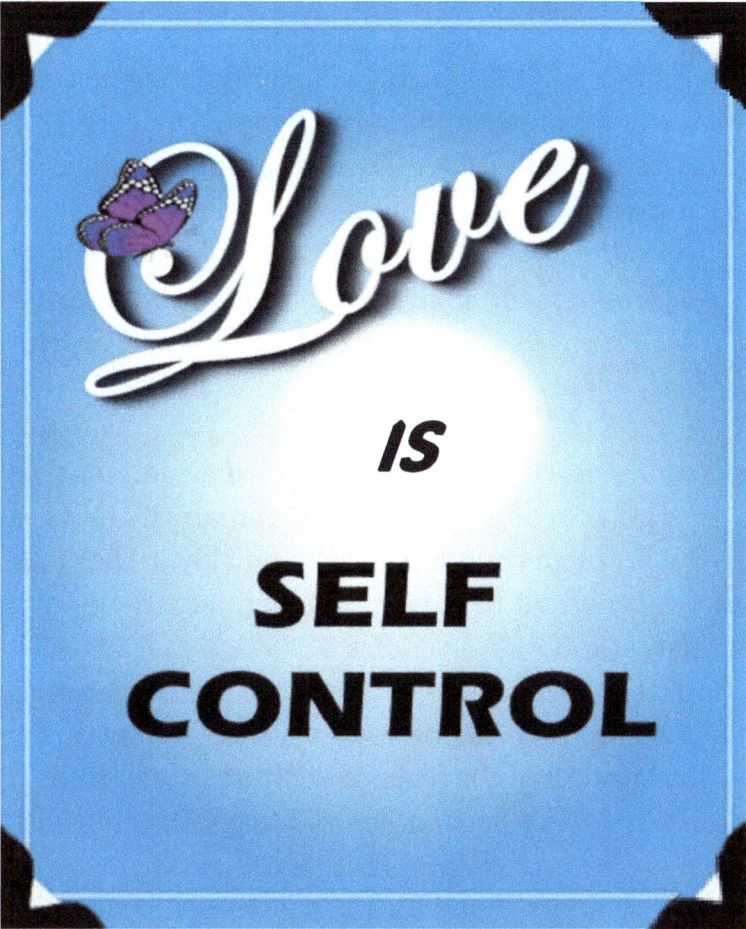

Love

IS

SELF CONTROL

The Gift of Self-Control

"Better a patient person than a warrior, one with self-control than one who takes a city." Proverbs 16:32 (NIV)

One definition of self-control is the ability to be in command of your behavior and restrain or inhibit your impulses. This can be especially challenging when the actions and reactions of those we love turn harmful and thoughtless.

My dear brothers and sisters, take note of this: Everyone should be quick to listen, slow to speak and slow to become angry,"
James 1:19 (NIV)

Illness and stress can lead to inappropriate actions from those we love and care for. It takes a lot of maturity and grace to recognize the problem cannot be solved quickly. In her telling the story, Forlorn Daughter has given each of us some sound advice in her last paragraph.

She found the fortitude to quit arguing and correcting her mother. She had to lay aside her own crushed feelings and thoughts. Forlorn Daughter realized it didn't matter in the long run; her job was to love her mother and to give her the best care possible.

When we're stressed, self-control tends to fly out the window. It takes wisdom and discipline to recognize and meet our own needs as we care for others. In Nancy's story, she offers two positive things she did to relieve stress as her mother's needs changed drastically. I am quite sure committing to leaving to be with friends for three hours each week was traumatizing at first.

Nancy also used her God-given ability to write poems as a way of releasing her feelings. (Even if you don't think you are a writer, you can feel relief from stress by writing out prayers to the Lord in a small journal or spiral notebook and leave that day's problems with Him.)

"No temptation has overtaken you except what is common to mankind. And God is faithful; he will not let you be tempted beyond what you can bear. But when you are tempted, he will also provide a way out so that you can endure it." 1 Corinthians 10:13 (NIV)

~Susie

The Story I Couldn't Tell

"Be kind and compassionate to one another, forgiving each other, just as in Christ God forgave you." Ephesians 4:32 (NIV)

My mother was slowly slipping into dementia. Initially, we guesstimated that she was confused only twenty percent of the time. As time passed and her congestive heart failure worsened, her mind was not her own about seventy percent of the time. Our clues included Mom using dish soap as oil for homemade bread, plus almost burning the house down when she forgot to turn off a propane stove and burnt the meat in the pan.

My sister and I agreed we should take her to a gerontologist with the hope there was a medication that would slow down the process of her memory loss, but first... Mom would have to be convinced to go – no easy task.

Mom reluctantly agreed to go to the doctor, but she and I made the hour-long journey to the doctor's office in near silence. She was visibly upset and tight-lipped. My sister met us at the doctor's office. As we talked with the doctor, I observed Mother getting madder and madder, pinching her lips together and grunting from time to time.

My sister was telling the doctor all the details for our visit when suddenly Mom had an outburst, screaming that the entire doctor's visit was my fault. Then, angrily, she reared back with her hand fully extended and slapped my face, making me almost fall from the chair. I left the meeting trying to keep it together, but it hurt both physically and mentally.

We never went back to the doctor. Her remaining years were a struggle for all of us. Mom wasn't my mother for many days in those last years. If she had been herself that day, I know she would never have hit me. Dementia and memory loss can cause people to do things outside their everyday routines.

I stopped correcting her and arguing about what truths were right before her. It was futile to think it would make a difference. To love her, I had to lay aside my feelings and thoughts and remember she was a woman who only wanted the best for her family all her life. Her memories were hers alone. They may have been scrambled memories with wrong names and blended stories, but it didn't matter. My job was to love her to the end.

~Forlorn Daughter

That's Not My Mama

"I have told you these things, so that in me you may have peace.
In this world you will have trouble. But take heart!
I have overcome the world." John 16:33 (NIV)

In June of 2015, Mother came to live with me. She was not steady on her feet and the doctor said she could no longer live alone; too much of a fall risk. My two brothers and their wives all had forty-hour-a-week jobs. Being the only daughter and already retired, I gladly took on the task of caregiver. My husband, also retired, was a pillar of help to me.

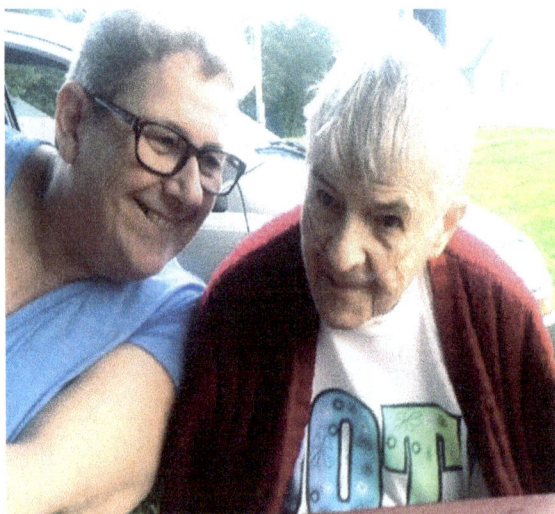

When she first came to live with us, it was like a vacation for her. She did not have to cook meals, do laundry or worry about writing checks to pay bills. She went shopping with me, we went out to eat and she could take care of her hygiene needs.

As time went by, her eyesight and hearing weakened, and her memory began to fail. Some days she wanted to pack and go home. She forgot my home was her home now. She became verbally abusive. I was going through an emotional trauma and needed a distraction. So, I spent one afternoon each week playing cards with friends for three hours.

I did most of my grieving months before her death as she was a shell of my mom, mind gone and very rarely speaking - just staring off into space. Poetry was my outlet to get my feelings out.

That's Not My Mama

Ninety years have taken its toll
Memories forgotten
eyes grew dim to nothing
and she became nearly deaf.
She got on the dementia train
which was the biggest curse yet.
She went into a long dark tunnel
and she never came out.
Dementia I hate you.
You stole my mother,
and I can't get her back.

Our Physician's Assistant asked us about getting some help in the house, specifically Hospice. My husband and I discussed this, but we didn't think we needed help. A few weeks before her death, however, we decided to ask Hospice for help. It was such a freeing experience. No longer did I fuss at her to eat or get dressed or get out of bed. I no longer felt guilty for not doing what I thought was right. It was her time to do what her body needed to do.

~Nancy LaChance

An Encouraging Word

"The Lord himself goes before you
and will be with you;
he will never leave you
nor forsake you.
Do not be afraid;
do not be discouraged."

Deuteronomy 31:8 (NIV)

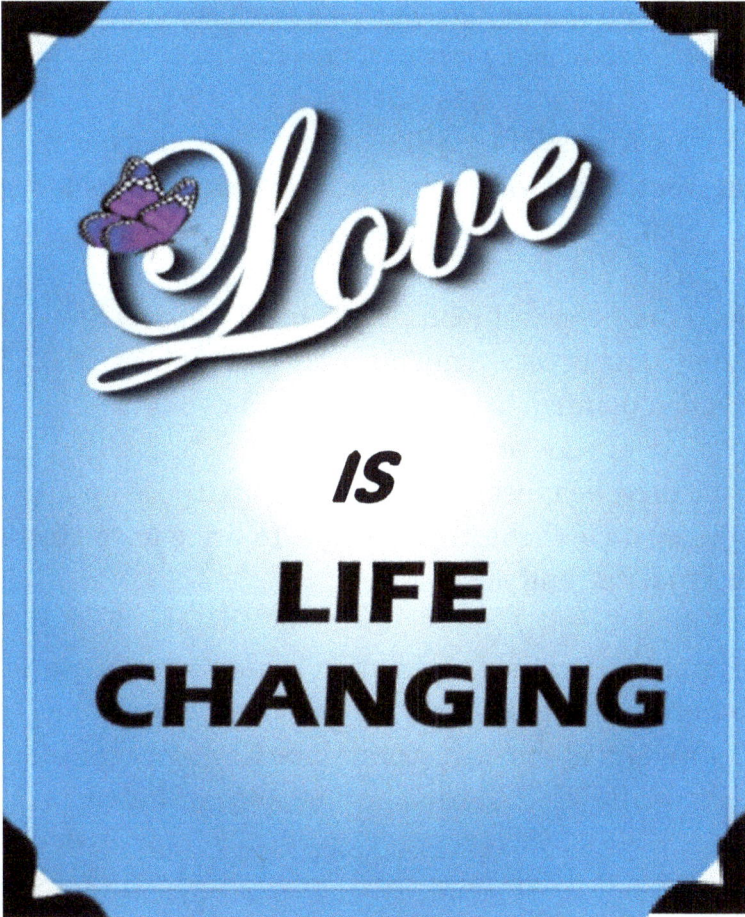

Love

IS

LIFE

CHANGING

Change is Inevitable

"Set your minds on things above, not on earthly things."
Colossians 3:2 (NIV)

"Many are the plans in a person's heart, but it is the Lord's purpose that prevails." Proverbs 19:21 (NIV)

If I were to describe my life from birth to this day in one word, it would have to be "change". Of course, there is the physical change we each must go through as we grow from birth and diapers to old age and ... Well, let's not go there!

The more I connect with people in all walks of life, one fact rings true. Most of us are not entering our senior years doing what we had planned to do with our lives.

If we are to believe that God is with us always, that He never leaves us, then we must believe He has a purpose for every bump along the way. He orchestrates events to bring us to His plan as we learn to listen and obey.

Deanna's life-changing moment came when she was given permission to turn the caregiving role over to someone else. Dorothy reveals in the next stories how having hospice care for her husband drew her to become a hospice volunteer.

~Susie

Why Are You Here?

"Fear not, for I am with you; be not dismayed, for I am your God; I will strengthen you, I will help you, I will uphold you with my righteous right hand." Isaiah 41:10 (ESV)

Two years ago, my mom was diagnosed with advanced bile duct cancer. She wanted to go home from the hospital and just be with her family and her puppies. So, we took her home.

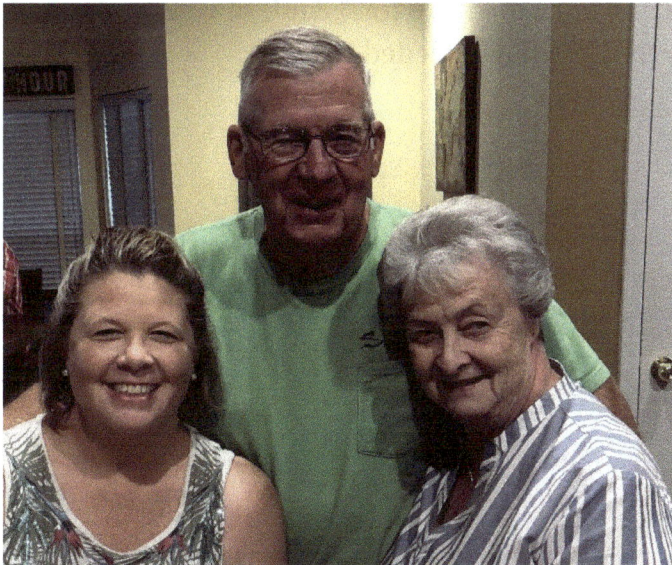

I am a registered nurse. There are no other nurses or healthcare workers in our family. I felt the weight of having to know all the right medical things to do to take care of Mom. I needed to take care of her *and* my family.

When the time came that we needed to start giving Mom medicine to keep her comfortable, the daughter in me loved her so and didn't want to let her go. I wanted her to stay awake; I wanted to visit with and love on her. At the same time, I also wanted to grieve this eminent loss. But as a nurse for many years, the nurse's hat never completely comes off. So, you stay strong. You are the one who needs to give her the medicines, change her bed, her gown, feed her, and take care of all that she needs. So much pressure!

The second day after we called hospice in, God sent this amazing nurse who knew right away I was conflicted. I was struggling to keep it together. A short time after her arrival, without a word, she helped me reposition Mom in her bed. Then, from across the bed, she took my hands and looked me in the eye. She lovingly said, "I'm giving you permission to be her daughter. You don't have to be her nurse, that's what I am here for." And, of course, we had a good cry. That was exactly what I needed to hear.

~Deanna Lane

Dorothy's Personal Experience

"I can do all things through Christ who strengthens me."
Philippians 4:13 (NKJV)

My husband, Steve, our cocker spaniel, Tex, and I received hospice care in our home in 2008. St. John's Hospice Care became our support system, thanks to Steve's compassionate doctor who understood what was happening and how to help us.

In the 1960's Steve had been gravely injured when serving our country in the U.S. Navy. After many years of surgeries, therapies and treatments, he learned how to manage several disabling conditions. We met, fell in love, and married. We soon found that our married life revolved around his disabilities. He asked me to promise never to put him in a nursing home. I promised because it was important to him. Ten years before Steve's passing, he suffered a high above-the-knee amputation because of uncontrollable osteomyelitis (a bone infection). In addition, he had a broken neck that hadn't healed properly and many other medical issues. He became a 100% disabled veteran; we coped as best we could with his worsening medical conditions. When he asked me to renew my promise to care for him at home, I did.

Thank God for hospice, even though the initial days of getting on service were overwhelming. Strangers came and went; I was given paperwork I couldn't focus on, but signed anyway. Deliveries of medical equipment and supplies required the rearrangement of possessions and furniture. When the hospital bed arrived, our volunteer fire department, with care and respect, settled Steve in our living room while they took our bed apart and removed it from our home. They set up the hospital bed and moved him back into our bedroom. During long nights when difficulties arose and I didn't know what to do, I was thankful for the Nurse on Call Service, which provided 24-hour support.

I slept on the floor near Steve's hospital bed so I would hear him if he needed me. Our dog Tex was delighted to find me on the floor, and honestly, I needed doggie cuddles as much as Tex needed mine. This was difficult for all of us.

Nurses and bath aides taught me how to care for my husband, who at 6'3" and over 200 pounds was helpless to help me. This military man, who expected everything to be exactly as he wanted it, was learning to let go. He had always known that leaving this earth was as much a part of life as his birth into it had been. His acceptance made it easier for me. Hospice helped him keep his dignity while giving us excellent care.

Each hospice worker who entered our home was respectful, kind, considerate, and loving. Only the Lord and I know how much I needed those visits. You see, Steve's disabilities isolated us from others. We had no family here and very few friends. Basically, hospice workers were my support system. They enabled me to keep my promise to my husband.

~ Dorothy Davidson

Dorothy Becomes a Hospice Volunteer

"Having then gifts differing according to the grace that is given to us, let us use them:" Romans 12:6a (NKJV)

Now, years later, with the volunteer training hospice provided and years of experience, I see I could have cared for Steve better than I did. At that time though, I was who I was, I knew much less than I do now. Then, I was overwhelmed with the situation, lack of sleep, and the coming loss. Now, I give myself grace for what I didn't know to do. I don't criticize the person I was then. God often gives us more grace than we give ourselves.

Eagerly I took the training that would allow me to help others. I found that many of our volunteers had been recipients of hospice services; we were glad to work together. For several months I volunteered in the office. There was paperwork to file, supplies to organize for nurses and aides, mailings to assemble, and at that hospice, there was a quilting and teddy bear ministry. I filled baskets with teddys decorated with bows, color coordinated them with baskets, quilts, and pillows; what a friendly welcome present to

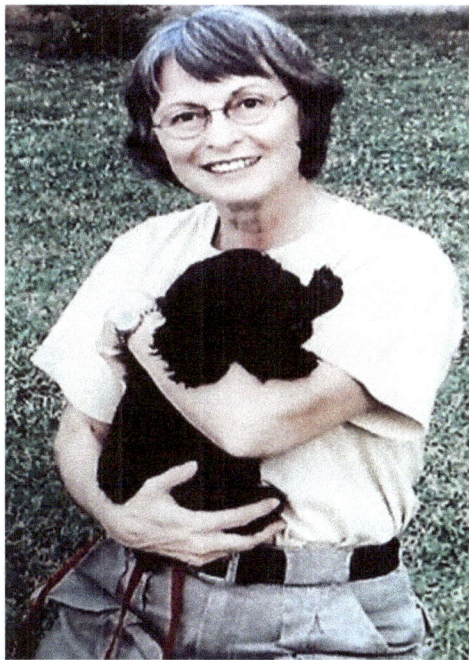

new families on hospice!

Advanced training in comfort care enabled me to visit families who requested a volunteer. I was not allowed to physically help patients, but there were many other ways to help.

I have sung hymns with patients, read to them from the Bible or a favorite book, written letters, played games, shared stories, made them laugh, distracted them from their situation. Sometimes they just needed a calming presence to hold their hand or to listen. I've tried to make a difference in this precious time when they are struggling with the diagnosis, saying goodbye to all they have loved, transitioning from one life to another.

My visits to homes enable caregivers to have free time to do what they choose: nap, walk, shop, go to the doctor, get their hair done. Caregivers also need someone to listen, someone without the emotional baggage of a family member. The key is to be receptive and perceptive, always holding information confidential. Our work with intake staff, nurses, aides, social workers, and chaplains makes us an effective team; our priority is family care and support.

When Steve and I received hospice services, there was no volunteer available to come to our country home, given the distance from Springfield. I vowed that as long as I could, I would go wherever there was need. I have been to families in Bolivar, Rogersville, and country homes that seemed a long way from civilization. I've also been to hospital rooms where I've had to wear protective gear for mutual safety. I have braved a dog bigger than I, who felt responsible for his charge and who eyed me with suspicion during my time there. (Later, I learned the couch I'd sat on was the big dog's bed.) I have laughed and cried with patients, family members, and staff. And, of course, I grieve when patients pass but I am so thankful to have been a part of their life, especially during this difficult time. While each patient and family have a different hospice experience, each volunteer does too. Our calling is challenging but incredibly rewarding.

Why do I do this? The Lord enabled me to have this ministry; it is my joy to do it. I have gained lifelong friends; I have even written a book with one dear family. There is satisfaction in helping people, of seeing their faces light up when I arrive, of joining in their laughter and their tears.

People have asked what I do with my retirement time. When I tell them, they often shake their heads and say they could not be with people who are dying. My answer is I'm privileged to visit people who are living. I pray before each visit that God will be with me, fill the home with His presence, and help me be what He needs me to be. Then we are ready to go make a difference in whatever way we can.

~ Dorothy Davidson

What is Hospice and How it can Help

Hospice comfort care focuses on quality of life, providing medical, emotional, and spiritual support to those who have received a terminal diagnosis. Treatment for the diagnosis is discontinued: no more tests and trips to the doctor. Instead, a hospice physician supervises a team of trained specialists who care for the patient and family in a variety of settings, from personal homes to memory care units. These specialists include nurses, home health care aids, social workers, spiritual support personnel, and volunteers.

~ Dorothy Davidson

Progress and Regression

A toddler has a fear of falling.
The elderly, too, fear falling.

As an infant is cutting teeth,
Older people are prone to losing theirs.

As an infant's vision increases,
Elderly people may suffer vision loss.

A child begins to babble,
As often do the elderly.

A baby grows a thicker head of hair
While some elderly began losing theirs.

A child's hearing brings understanding.
An older person's hearing brings confusion.

A baby will learn to sleep through the night.
Older people often have trouble sleeping.

A toddler gains bladder control.
The aging population may lose bladder control.

A young heart provides amazing energy.
The aged heart slows their body down.

The memory of a young child is like a thirsty sponge.
The memory of an older person is a daily battle.

~ Donna Barnes

An Encouraging Word

"For our light and momentary Troubles are achieving for us an eternal glory that far outweighs them all."

2 Corinthians 4:17 (NIV)

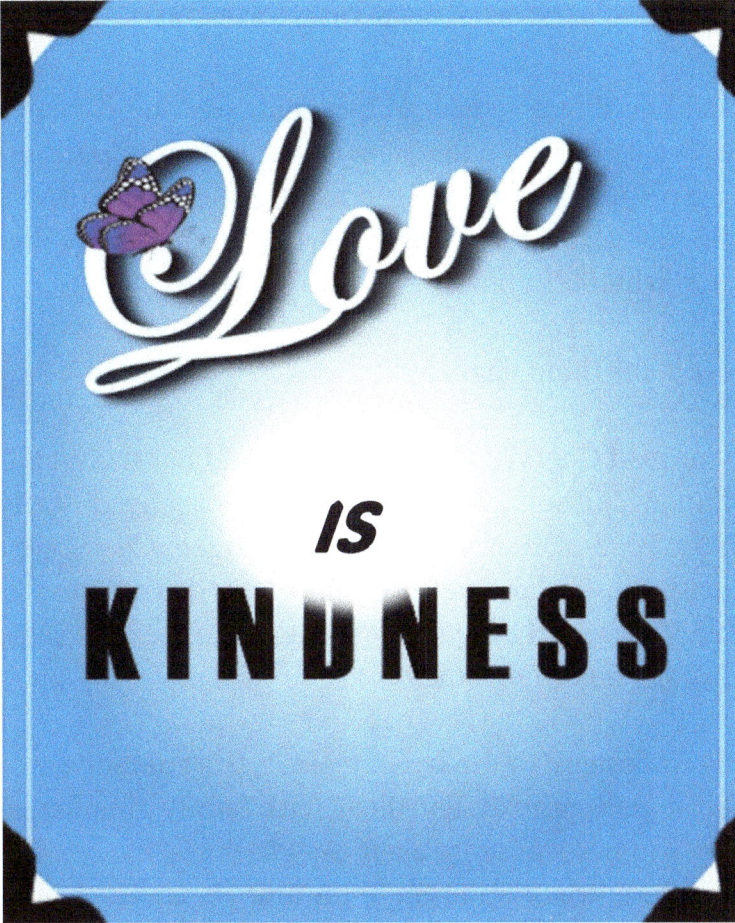

Love

IS

KINDNESS

Kindness Matters

"My children, our love should not be only words and talk. No, our love must be real. We must show our love by the things we do."
1 John 3:18 (ERV)

Biblical kindness is marked by generosity and concern for others without expecting praise or reward in return. It's going the extra mile when you are worn to a frazzle with no end in sight. Showing kindness and compassion is not simply the act of doing good when it's convenient.

Health issues cause our loved ones to behave in ways that make caring for them challenging.

As you read Cheryl's story, keep in mind her daily routine never changed, although her circumstances changed drastically through the years. Often, though weary herself, Cheryl would load Doug in the car and take him on a long drive to familiar places. This was good for each of them as they relived cherished memories of a healthier time.

Daily walking with the Lord, seeking His guidance as we make decisions is crucial. For those with family members close by, the decisions seem more clear. As Pauline and her family began to assess Ron's situation, it became apparent that he needed to spend his last days in his home. Watch for God's affirming miracles!

~Susie

Through It All

"Fear not, for I am with you; be not dismayed, for I am your God; I will strengthen you, Yes, I will help you, I will uphold you with My righteous right hand." Isaiah 41:10 (NKJV)

Twenty-year-old lovebirds, Cheryl Mallard and Douglas Gardner, wed in June 1971 in Kansas City, Missouri. From day one, they were devoted to each other and to the Lord and His will for their lives.

Thirteen years later their life's journey took a dramatic turn when Doug began experiencing serious health issues. Still facing each day with the Lord, they celebrated events such as no hospital visit for three months, then none for six months, then a couple of years with no hospital visits.

On a particular night of bowling, Doug became very ill. An alert friend insisted he be taken immediately to the emergency room. This most likely spared his life because we learned he suffered from a massive heart attack.

After several illnesses and surgeries, the Gardners moved to Buffalo, Missouri to help care for Cheryl's parents. Cheryl faced the task of moving her parents from the home they'd lived in for forty-five years. She took care of her parents' needs each morning and then turned her attention to Doug's needs.

Doug's health was also failing. Cheryl struggled with the decline in his health, as oxygen and a wheelchair were now necessary 24/7. This meant changing vehicles and adjusting schedules to meet the growing needs of her parents and her husband.

Due to her mother's stroke and her father's deteriorating health, Cheryl's parents were moved to a care facility. With both parents in the care facility, Cheryl and her brother began the task of preparing their homeplace to be put on the market. Cheryl says, *"We discovered that Mom had lots of 'hidden' things for us to do something with."*

Her folks' minivan was the perfect solution for Doug's increasing mobility needs. The timing was perfect. A wheelchair could easily be folded for transport, and the van could accommodate several tanks of oxygen for their many trips from Buffalo to Kansas City for Doug's growing medical needs.

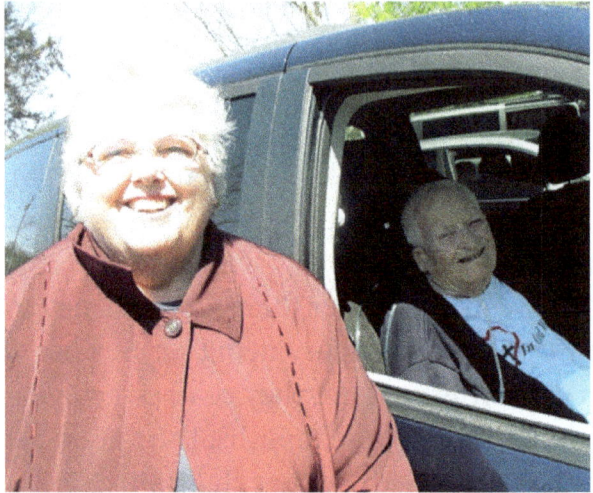

Cheryl's dad and Doug passed within six months of each other. Her mother was moved to the Baptist Home in Ozark, Missouri, where she lived two more years.

Cheryl's words- *"My pastor told me a couple of weeks after Doug died that I looked like I was getting some rest. My daily life for so many years had been caring for family. I had no idea how worn out I was. I guess 37 years of looking after him, and then my parents had taken their toll. The Lord knew, and He provided my daily needs. One thing about Doug... he never really complained about his disabilities. He served the Lord to the end. The marriage vows say, 'in sickness and in health' ... and that was a vow neither of us was going to break!"*

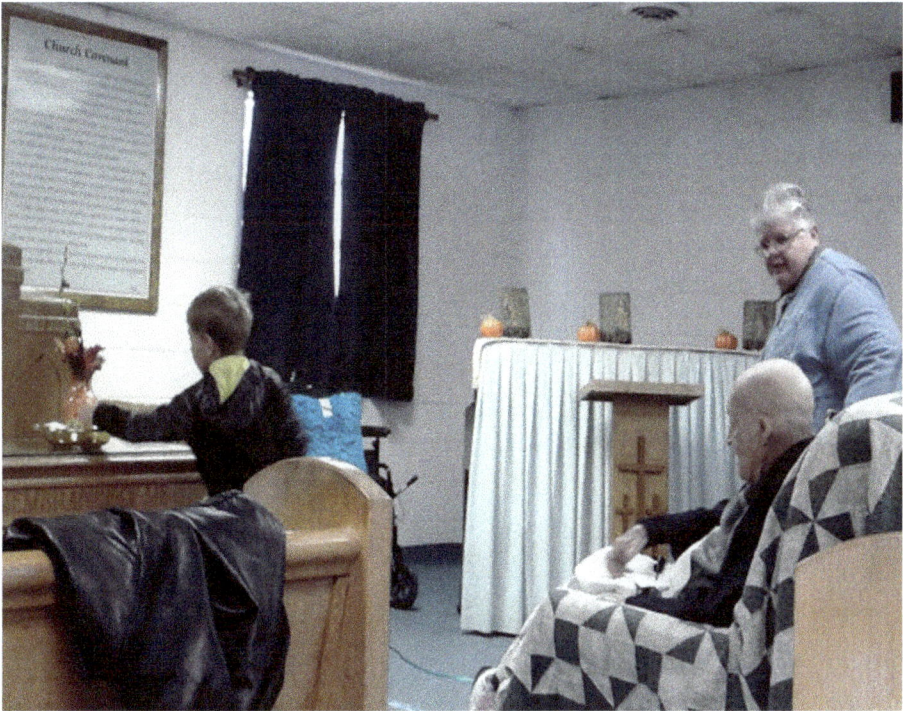

Amid her challenges, Cheryl continued to not only faithfully attend but also serve her church. The church had allowed a comfy recliner to be put into the sanctuary for her husband, Doug, so they could attend worship together. Cheryl taught Sunday School, served on committees, led mission endeavors, and was involved in association work. She also served her community by delivering commodities and caring for her neighbors' needs. Cheryl continues to serve the Lord in many capacities today.

~Cheryl Gardner as told to Susie Kinslow Adams

Home is Where the Heart Is

"Return to your home,
and declare how much God has done for you."
Luke 8:39 (ESV)

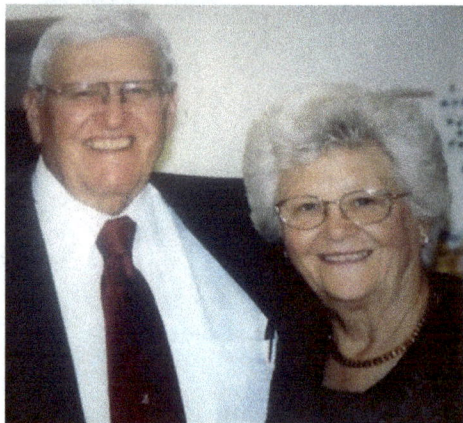

August 2020 – My husband, Ronald Lilley, was not feeling well. The home nurse came for her regular visit. She took Ron's vitals, which were not good. She told us he needed to go to the hospital. COVID was rampant... He was admitted. I could only see him for two hours a day.

Day 2 - His room was a mess, and he wasn't eating.

Day 3 - My daughter and I went to Outback Steak House and got him a steak, baked potato, and salad. He ate it all.

Day 4 - I was there when they brought his dinner. There was only a small hamburger patty on his plate. I asked the nurse, "Where is his food?" She said, "That's all he wanted." I was heartbroken. The doctor told me he needed to be moved to a skilled nursing facility. I wouldn't be able to see him for ten days... and then only through a glass window. Ron didn't want that – neither did I. "Do you want me to tell the doctor that we want to take you home?" He told me "Yes." I called the children to consult with them and they said, "Take him home."

Day 5 - He was dismissed this morning. He was so weak he couldn't walk. When we got home, our son-in-law and grandson were there to carry him into the house to his recliner.

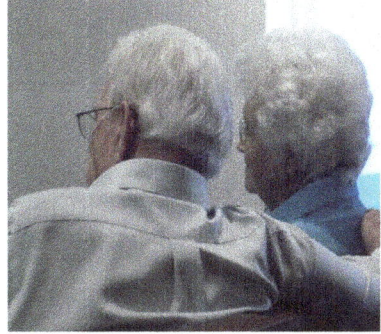

He rested for maybe two hours and then he got up by himself and walked to the bedroom to his bed. He was so happy to be back in his own surroundings; I was also happy to have him back at home.

Thank you, Jesus, for opening my eyes and allowing me to bring him home!

He is in his heavenly home now. I miss him so much but am thankful for so many great memories.

~ Pauline Lilley

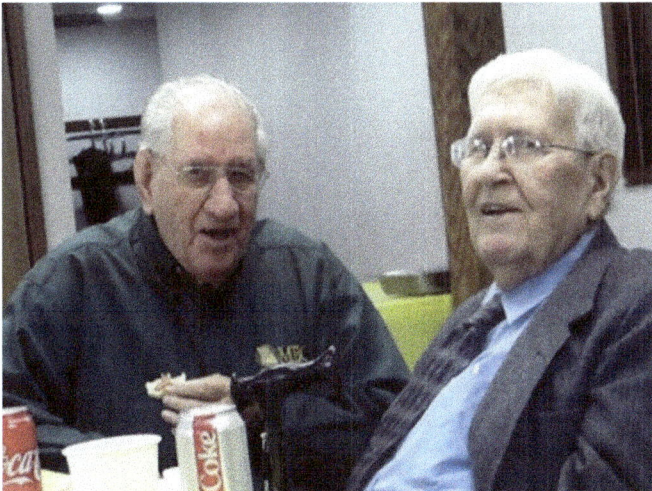

Director of Missions Russell Adams and Pastor Ronald Lilley were blessed to be in their own homes with family when God called them Home.

You Don't Lose Someone Just Once

You lose them over and over,
    sometimes many times a day.
When the loss, momentarily forgotten,
    creeps up,
    and attacks you from behind.
Fresh waves of grief as the realization hits home,

    they are gone.
      Again.

You don't just lose someone once,
    you lose them every time
 you open your eyes to a new dawn,
 and as you awaken,
so does your memory,
so does the jolting bolt of lightning
that rips into your heart,

    they are gone.
      Again.

Losing someone is a journey,
Not an on and off.
There is no end to the loss,
there is only a learned skill
      on how to stay afloat,
            when it washes over.

Be kind to those who are sailing this stormy sea,
      they have a journey ahead of them,
and a daily shock to the system
each time they realize,

      they are gone,
         Again.

You don't just lose someone once,
      you lose them every day,
         for a lifetime.

~Jeff Metcalf

An Encouraging Word

**"I lift up my eyes to the mountains
Where does my help come from?
My help comes from the Lord,
the Maker of heaven and earth."**

Psalm 121:1-2 (NIV)

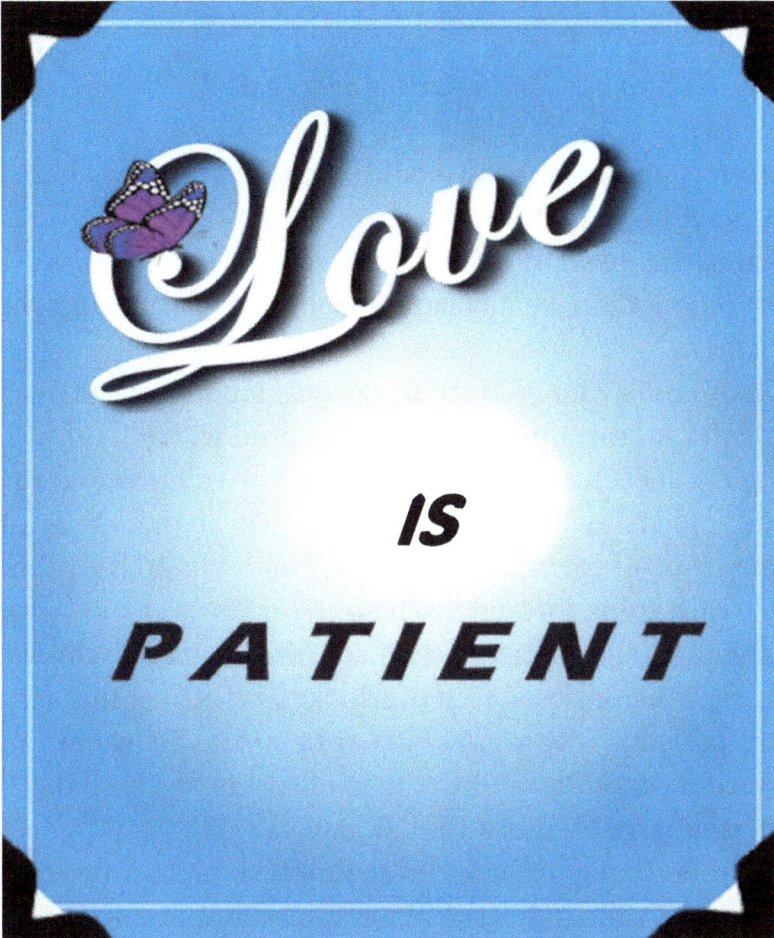

God Provides Patience

"And let us not get tired of doing what is right, for after a while we will reap a harvest of blessing if we don't get discouraged and give up."
Galatians 6:9 (TLB)

I appreciate the honesty of Joy and Cathy as they share their stories of caring for family members. When siblings and their families are involved, it certainly takes more patience and understanding than we have apart from our relationship with Jesus Christ.

When I took care of Mother, my only sibling was miles away. He did offer moral support and was pleased with whatever I chose to do in each situation. However, I often hungered to just sit down and visit with him face-to-face. Through no fault of their own, out-of-town siblings cannot understand the scope of what you are going through each day.

Indeed, it takes patience with others as you carry out your daily caregiving duties. Often overlooked is the fact that it also requires patience with yourself. We are mortal beings; we will make mistakes. As Joy and Cathy made decisions each day, they leaned heavily on the Lord for guidance.

Whether caring for another or simply living day by day in a sinful world, Psalm 5:3 is the prescription for patience and the remedy for all our needs.

"In the morning, Lord, You will hear my voice; In the morning I will present my prayer to You and be on the watch." Psalm 5:3 (NASB)

~Susie

Expect the Unexpected

"Now the God of patience and consolation grant you to be likeminded one toward another according to Christ Jesus:"
Romans 15:5 (KJV)

Our mother was a very active lady before a stroke took its toll. By very active I mean my petite 4' 9" mother daily RAN out the front door down a tall step out to the mailbox 95 feet away.

In 2015, my 80-year-old mother had a stroke and fell in her home. I didn't discover her for eleven hours, although I lived next door. (She had been sick over the weekend and had told me she was going to brush her teeth and go back to bed. Mother said she would be fine by herself and encouraged me to go home and watch football with my husband. So, I left.)

She had a stroke while she was brushing her teeth. She managed to crawl out of her bathroom and down a narrow hallway to the kitchen wall phone. She struggled to knock the receiver off the hook, until she realized that she wouldn't be able to dial even if she had the receiver. She then tried to get to the living room where she had left her cordless phone. I found her the next morning when she didn't answer my normal morning phone call.

Mother was in a nursing home for about four months and when she came home, she had very little use of her right hand, it had atrophied. She was able to walk but with a walker. She needed help dressing and undressing but was able to go to the bathroom and cook food in the microwave that was ready for her to eat. All that fell on me or my daughters, sister-in-law or nieces to do. I scheduled all of it.

Many times, I felt my brothers were clueless. It was frustrating that they did not understand how frail Mom was. One lived in Florida, one lived in New Mexico, and one hid himself in his work, though he lived ten miles away. The one who did understand was scared and although he refused to physically help with her care, his wife did help when she could.

My husband and I were fortunate to live right next door so Mother could stay in her home a little over three years before she passed away. We installed a nursery monitor in her bedroom and ours and got her a Life Alert necklace, which she wore 24/7.

I am so thankful for those who did help me! It truly takes a village. BUT the village needs to be in place long before you need to use it! Trust is essential! It doesn't come overnight.

~Joy Bowser

It Takes a Village

"Two are better than one because they have a good reward for their toil. For if they fall, one will lift up his fellow. But woe to him who is alone when he falls and has not another to lift him up!"
Ecclesiastes 4:9-10 (ESV)

Our family has been blessed to be followers of Jesus and have His influence and understanding as we jointly cared for our parents and their ever-changing needs. Because of our desire to obey the Bible's commandments, we have been able to work together within our situation to assist Daddy's journey into the next life.

My youngest brother and his wife were still working but live within fifteen miles of mom and dad's. My husband and I and my other siblings and their spouses were retired. I want to take a moment to praise our spouses. Life would have been very difficult if our spouses had not supported and pitched in to help whenever and wherever needed.

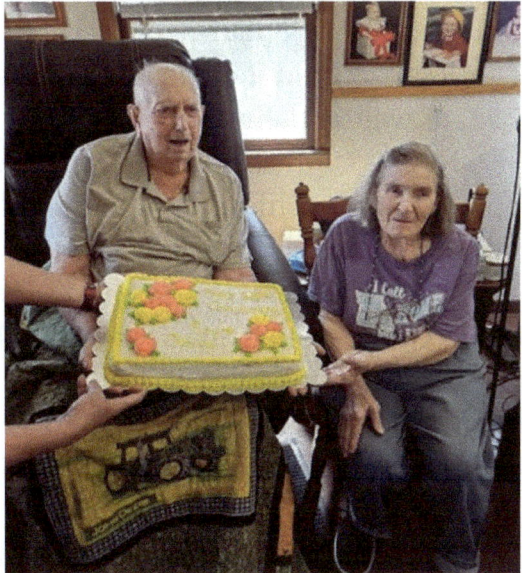

In mid-November, Dad was diagnosed with cancer. He was 85 years old and had congestive heart failure, COPD, and the beginnings of renal failure. Dad had two options: go home on hospice or take chemo for a probable cure.

Most of the family agreed with Mother. We wanted Dad to choose hospice hoping they could keep him alive longer. But it was Dad's decision. I was neutral since I had been down the cancer treatment road with my husband and understood that the patient and his or her attitude was very much the determining factor in how well they did on any plan of treatment. (Dad told me toward the end of his life that he was in so much pain with the cancer, but he wanted to live as long as he could.)

In the time leading up to the chemo treatments, we planned who would stay with Mom and Dad the few days after the treatments. Because my husband had gone through chemo treatments, this task fell to me. My sister, Anna, and I had already been sharing our parents' doctor appointments for about five years. Now that Dad had so many prescriptions and my sister had been a pharmacy tech, she took Dad, and I took Mom. Our duties would include any medical needs that "our parent" had, as well as their medicines.

NOTE: In the beginning, we tried taking turns with doctor appointments. This did not work well because we would disagree on treatment and treatment plans or the doctor, etc. We quickly realized it was best if we each were responsible for one parent's care. (Occasionally, one of us would have to cover for the other, but we understood the ground rules, so we didn't complain about what the other did.) We began this routine when they only needed occasional help, so it was easy to keep up now that full-time care was required.

Anna had been getting their medicines, filling up their weekly dispensers, and paying their bills for a while before this happened. Since she had been department head and ran her own business, she worked with people well. Therefore, we agreed as a family on what we needed from our employees and let her do the hiring.

The people we hired were informed that our parents were to be their boss. Duties in order of importance were:

1. See to the immediate needs of our parents.
2. See that all medicines were given.
3. Cook meals for them.
4. Clean house.

We also expressed that we did not expect them to hurt themselves by lifting our parents. They were to let us know if anything was wrong, and we would remedy it. We were blessed with women who were Christians, and with one exception, there was no drama, and they all got along.

There were checklists of chores that needed to be done at the end of each shift, if Mom or Dad wasn't too sick and all their immediate needs were taken care of:

1. All dishes were to be washed
2. All trash cans emptied & taken down to the dumpster
3. Laundry done
4. Beds made and everything tidied up

Then they were to do any other chores as deemed necessary by Mom or Dad. (Sometimes Dad would send them to town to get a special meal.)

Having each person responsible for their own shift's mess kept problems down.

In the beginning, we had a pass-down notebook: Each person was to record anything different, like changes in the skin or tiredness, what they ate, BM (Bowel Movement), Blood sugars, or an added medication that was needed due to illness, like a cold or UTI that occurred during their shift.

As Dad's situation worsened, it was harder to pick out anything that the next shift needed to be aware of in the pass-down notebook. We added a medication record sheet so the next shift could see at a glance the medications and times given. As needs changed, it was expanded to record BM, blood sugar and blood pressure when it was an issue. This became more important as Dad needed additional medication on a timed schedule and his and even Mom's vitals became an issue.

A current list of phone numbers was posted on the cabinet for all to see. This was vital for our family and for our helpers. Early in the process, we called a family meeting among us kids in a place where we wouldn't be interrupted. A big help in this initial meeting was a written agenda. We each compiled a list of things that had to be done, which kept us on topic as we made decisions. At the end of the meeting, everyone had a good sense of their jobs and what they needed to accomplish and by what time. *We also were able to more fully vent our worries and sometimes our frustrations... In that, we comforted each other.*

As the need arose, my sister, brother and I took time to come together for meetings when we faced issues needing a decision. This was done away from Mom and Dad. It might have seemed underhanded, but we would usually have to talk to my parents later about our discussion. In these meetings, we would choose which of us was to talk to Mom and Dad. These things often fell to my little brother because Dad was more apt to listen to him regarding just about anything - especially money issues.

There were several things that Dad was unwilling to budge on, including control of his finances and money sources. But as time went on, he began to turn things over to us kids, mainly because he could no longer physically show up and sign checks, easily access his retirement fund, etc.

He also refused to sign a DNR. This concerned us because he was never going to get better. Still, we did not push, but we prayed that we would not be put in that situation, and we just put it in the Lord's hands. We did not have to worry about this in the end, but I know many have not been as fortunate.

Dad had been struggling to breathe but he refused to go to the hospital. So, we told him after Christmas, he was going. He seemed to brighten in the hospital and was doing well. About the fourth day he had what is called 'Hospital Delirium.' This is a hallucination that occurs mostly in older hospital patients with breathing problems. They believe they experienced something horrible, and it is real to them. There is no talking them out of it, and you will only stress them if you treat their hallucination as something less than the truth. His doctor would have preferred to keep him for a couple more days, but the stress of what Dad thought he saw was worse on him than going home.

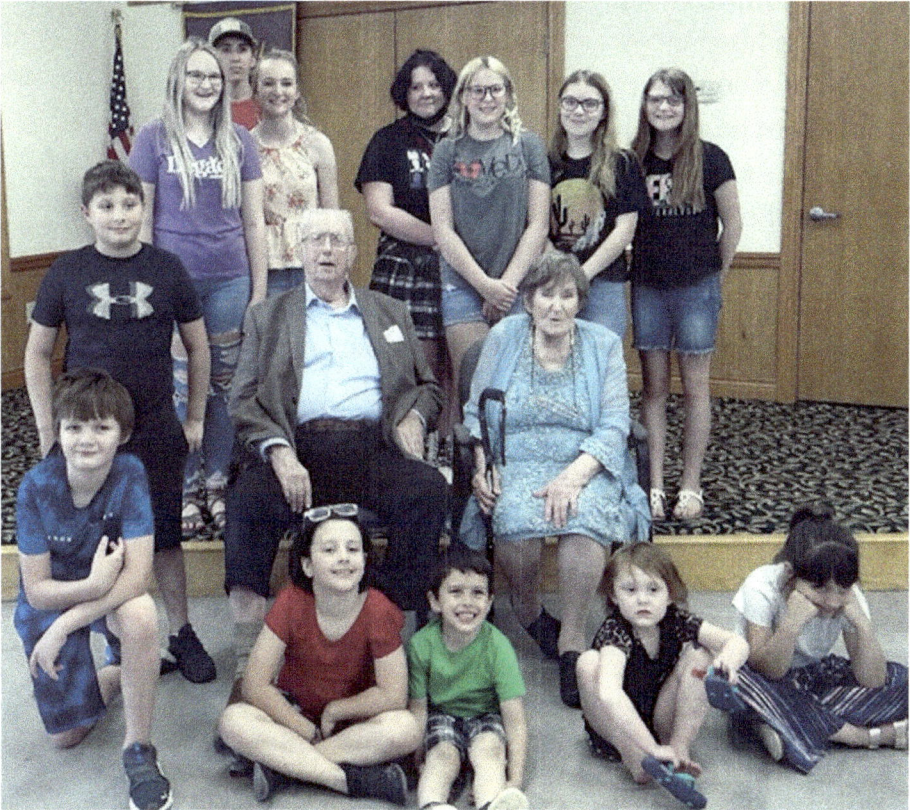

When Dad came home, he could no longer stand without being lifted. None of us could physically lift him out of bed onto a potty chair. We had to use a lift to get him out of bed. We were afraid of this in the hospital and had the forethought and finances to buy a queen-sized adjustable bed so that Mom could sleep with him like they normally did, and placed it in the living room. (This was hard on Mom, but we felt her sleeping in a recliner beside a hospital bed would have been worse for her.)

Once he had to be diapered, I think that was it. His body was just worn out. His COPD was getting the best of him, his kidneys were failing, and his heart was beating its last. Because he couldn't stand, we couldn't take him to his post-hospital doctor's visit. Without that visit, he couldn't get his medications, so he was put on hospice.

Not all people have the physical, spiritual, or financial resources to handle the final stages of life. We had resisted hospice until the end because we were equipped as a family to take care of our dad's needs. We had a strong network from a year of Dad's gradual dying, but when the need for help came hospice was fantastic. They gave us the tools to make our task of helping Dad to the other side much easier on us and on him.

In the last forty-eight hours, our help came down with the flu and my sister and I had to administer the medications. Hospice gives you excellent instructions on what to expect and we were able to read and understand what was going on. Our family has been no stranger to death and so we were able to handle it. That being said, my father passed so easily. I've heard the horror stories of many people whose loved ones did not. So be sure and have some outside help. Call your church, friends, neighbors, whomever. And don't be ashamed to send them to the hospital for help.

My aunt and uncle didn't want anyone, including the grandchildren, to help them or Mom and Dad when my Dad's mother passed away. On a day I stopped by after church to see what was needed, Grandma had been left alone. My mother was in the adjoining bedroom, crying. My dad and uncle (grandma's sons) were out in the yard crying. I think my aunt was in the living room crying. My brother, his wife and I were with my grandmother when she passed from this life into the next. Mother, through her tears, told me to never try to care for someone dying without having people around to help you.

In the case of my mother, we will move. It's what's best for her and she knows there will be no peace where she lives.

It has been about a month now and she is starting to feel much deeper emotions. It is important to help the parent who remains to socialize with people frequently.

We are going to go to a Widow's conference. We have Bible study at some time through the day, and we visit at night after "Wheel of Fortune." *Remember to laugh.*

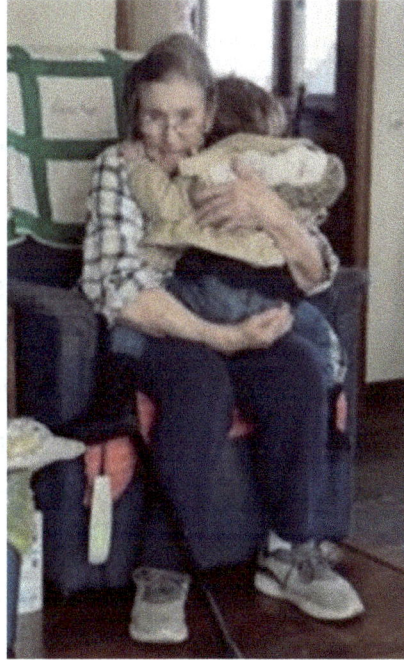

~ Cathy VanDruff

An Encouraging Word

"I will instruct you
and teach you
in the way you should go;
I will counsel you
with my loving eye on you."

Psalm 32:8 (NIV)

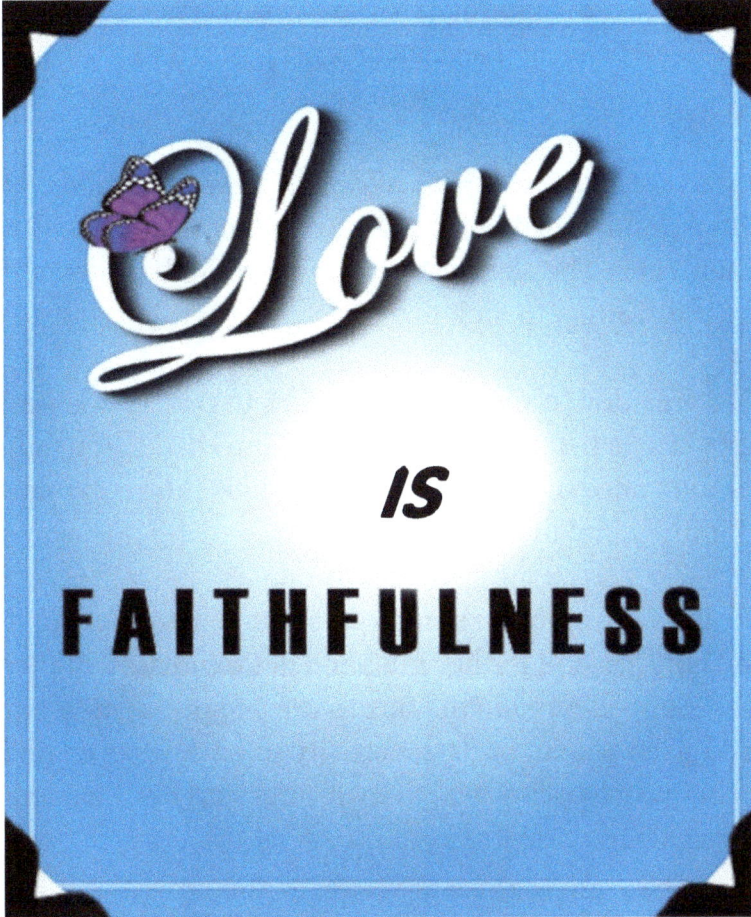

Love

IS

FAITHFULNESS

Great is His Faithfulness

"Because of the Lord's great love we are not consumed, for his compassions never fail. They are new every morning; great is your faithfulness." Lamentations 3:22-23 (NIV)

God's faithfulness to His children knows no bounds. His faithfulness and love do not mean we will not suffer health issues and other trials. The slightest headache can pull us down if our eyes are not trained to look up.

It's refreshing to read Ruth's praises to God as she walks through various health issues. We are reminded through her note of the importance of caring one for another. I'm so thankful for God's family in my life.

Our lives are complex; memories can be fleeting. Sondra's love and compassion for her husband are expressed in the many ways she stepped outside the box to create special moments for him. God used a neighbor's generosity to give her even another interesting way to provide activity for her and her husband to enjoy together.

As I write this, I cannot help but think about those times in my life when I cared for someone: my mother, my brother, my cousin, my husband, and a friend. Often my thoughts were on meeting the immediate physical need without considering the deeper spiritual need. Good memories are food for the soul and lift the spirit of both the one being cared for and the caregiver.

As you personally think of the faithfulness of God in your life, consider writing down some memories you cherish. If only for yourself, you will find it a healing balm for your weary soul.

"Forever, O Lord. Your word is settled in heaven. Your faithfulness endures to all generations; You established the earth, and it abides."
Psalm 119:89-90 (NKJV)

"Do not withhold your mercy from me, LORD; may your love and faithfulness always protect me."
Psalm 40:11 (NIV)

~Susie

Best Birthday Ever

"Praise the Lord! Praise the Lord, O my soul! I will praise the Lord as long as I live; I will sing praises to my God while I have my being."
Psalm 146:1-2 (ESV)

Friends have been so faithful to pray, message, call, bring food, provide transportation – there's a long list of creative ways they have blessed our family. I applaud and thank them! Each touch has blessed my heart.

I sent a message to my friends giving them the latest update on my health. The news was as follows: "The congestive heart failure diagnosis in my recent ER/hospitalization has been reevaluated. We are now told by Mercy Cardiology that there is NO evidence of heart failure." I have great confidence in the Mercy Care Team, and they were wonderful at every step. *We're celebrating!* Spread the wonderful news. Thank you, God, and thanks to Mercy, and to you – our wonderful prayer partners.

I reminded them I was in the middle of chemo last year when I fell and broke two ribs. Cancer recovery procedures had to take a backseat for a short while, but soon I was to start both chemo and immunotherapy. However, my oncologist gave me the option of doing only immunotherapy. If my lab numbers went back up, I could add the chemo regimen at any time. That was wonderful news for me! Last year, Chemo was difficult and hugely expensive. I so rejoiced at this option. (Happy Birthday to me!) I had no adverse effects from the infusion except a little wakefulness that first night-thinking and rejoicing and wishing/praying good news such as this for several people I had seen at the Cancer Center during my treatment.

I cringed at writing a long message about my health and had been silent about the journey. So many patients I came across in the Cancer Center have heavier, life-changing, even hope-robbing issues.

A load was lifted!

Thanks to my beloved and most powerful God. Thank you, my unmatched hands, on the task of making me well. I thank my generous God who has showered me with healing, an amazing medical Care Team and a multitude of caring and loving friends. My good and faithful friends did well, and I love them so much and pray that even on this very day they will be rewarded by Him for their care for our family. I love you, dear ones.

Best birthday ever!!

~ Ruth Marshall

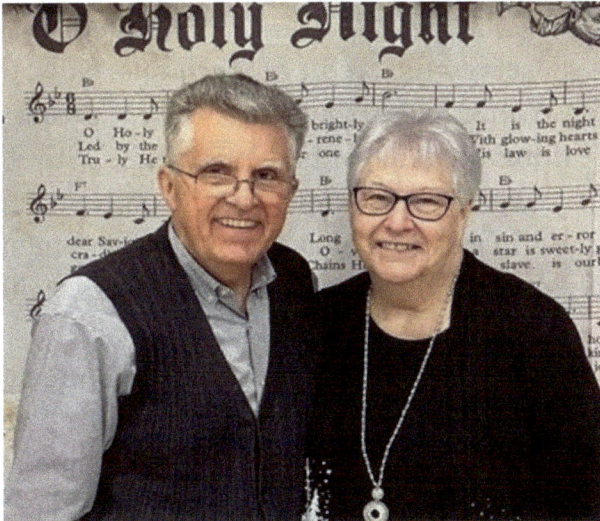

But Yesterday's Gone

"For we are of but yesterday, and know nothing, because our days on earth are a shadow." Job 8:9 (KJV)

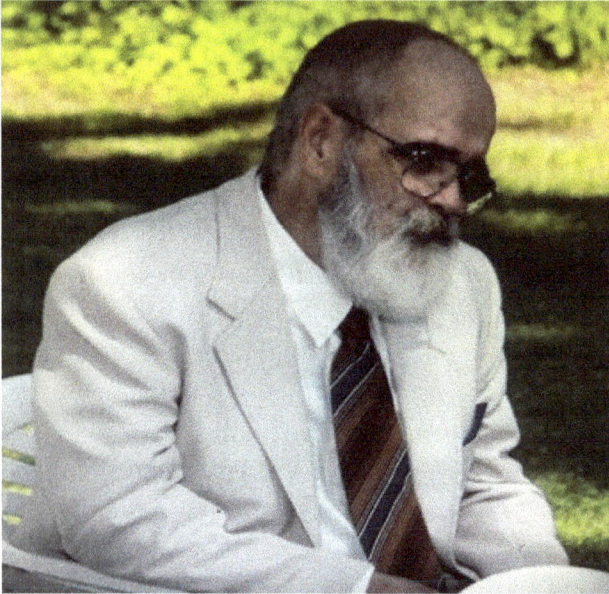

He couldn't remember what he had for breakfast or which of our sons came to see him yesterday, but he could tell me in precise detail when and where we met fifty-six years prior. He could recount with incredible accuracy the good times we had as well as the bad, and who deserved the credit for each one. Now, the doctor was telling me Walter had Alzheimer's. How was that possible? That was one thing I had never had experience with. I knew the symptoms, but what I didn't know was the daily struggles he would encounter in carrying on a conversation, remembering where he had left his wallet or recognizing me, his wife of fifty-four years.

As the struggles grew harder, I noticed how much happier he was when we were talking about the past. He didn't mind the same stories over and over. Matter of fact, he seemed to enjoy the repetition. I tried to think of something that would entertain him when I had other chores that had to be done. I turned to the trusty Internet! Everyone I could think of, especially people who had known him in the past, got an e-mail from me. I asked for letters, pictures, cards and especially funny stories about him. Believe me when I tell you, there was an abundance of those.

Emails started pouring in. I printed each one and put them, along with the cards, pictures and letters into an album, with each having its own dedicated page. I kept it on his bedside table so he could get to it anytime he wanted. He spent hours reading them and was so content in "that other lifetime."

Talking about the past with him started me thinking about his most prized possession as a young man. There was no doubt! It was his sharp red and white fifty-seven Chevy that we had taken on a date so many times. Again, I consulted the internet and found a picture that could have been *his* Chevy. I printed an eight by ten photo and put it into his album. I also found one exactly like the fifty-nine Chevy I had during the same time and added it to the collection. He looked at his album and studied each contribution, sometimes several times a day.

What man doesn't derive pleasure in watching a woman doing vigorous work? That was alright. I was willing to stoop to that level. Occasionally, I drove our car into the yard and parked it just outside his window. I had not manually washed a car in years, but I hadn't forgotten how. That gave me a chance to get out of the house for a while, saved a little money and entertained him. With his bedroom window raised, we could talk while I toiled and sweated. He always enjoyed making little comments such as "You missed a spot," but he never failed to comment on how good the car looked when I finished it.

That project went well, so I decided to try a new one. I built a raised bed garden about twenty-five feet from his window. I bought tomato plants; onion sets and various vegetables. I brought some seed, soil and pots inside and let him plant some starters. There was squash, zucchini and peppers. He enjoyed talking about "our" garden. He really enjoyed watching it grow, and the food from it tasted better to him than if I had bought it from a store.

When the gardening season was almost over, a friend told me they had more chickens than they needed. That presented new possibilities. I bought a chicken house kit and assembled it right at the end of the garden where Walt could still watch me from his window. I asked him to name our new pets. It took him several days, but he enjoyed it - there was Blondie, Annie, Katie, and Charlotte. Their eggs were good, and plentiful.

A large dry-erase board on the wall at the foot of Walter's bed made a good place to write notes, jokes or reminders for him. Even the date and day of the week gave him something to

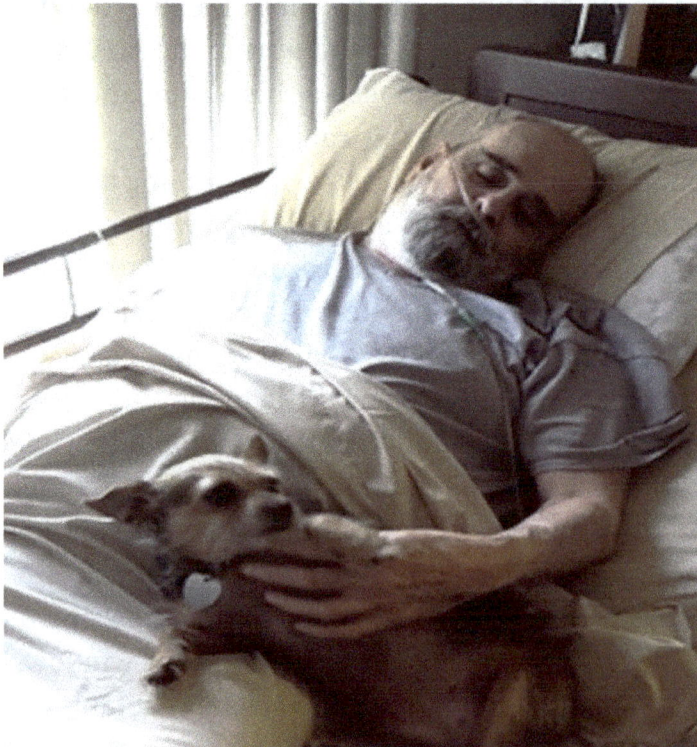

think about. I drew sketches which he always found amusing. I don't know why! Sometimes he didn't notice for a couple of days when I changed them, but sometimes he laughed or commented on them several times a day as if he had never seen them.

Walter could hold onto his puppy when he could hardly do anything else on his own. Often he would brave a smile as he commented: "I always have a little Hope." The dog was aptly named "Hope".

Now that Walter is gone, I have too much spare time. I often think of things I could and should have done, but I suppose that would always be the case. I miss him every day of my life, but I'm thankful for the good times God gave us, and for the knowledge and strength to do a few things to make his last days a little more pleasant.

~Sondra Gray

An Encouraging Word

**"Whatever you do,
work at it with all your heart,
as working for the Lord,
not for human masters,
since you know
that you will receive an inheritance
from the Lord as a reward.
It is the Lord Christ you are serving."**

Colossians 3:23-24 (NIV)

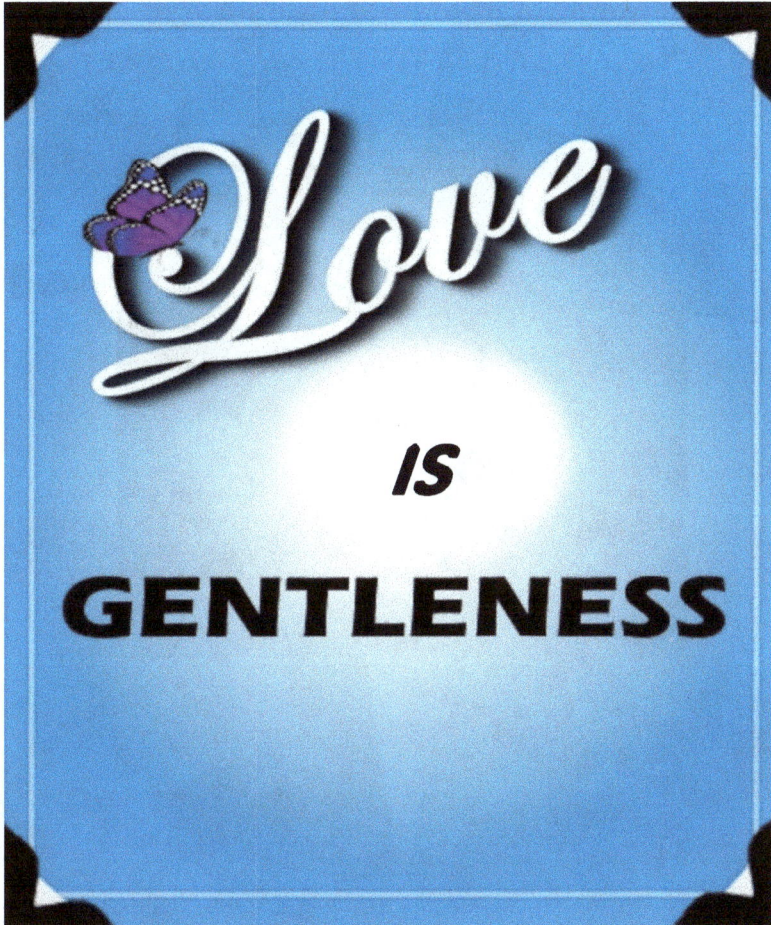

Love

IS

GENTLENESS

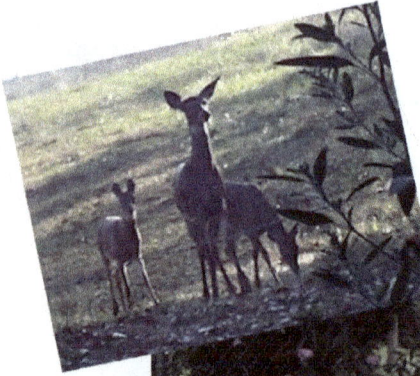
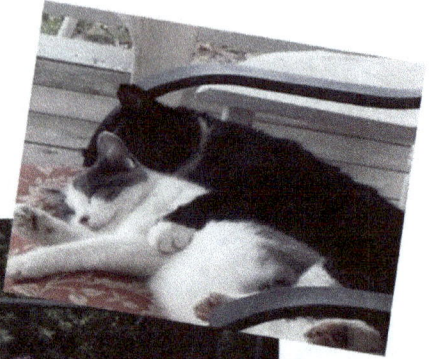
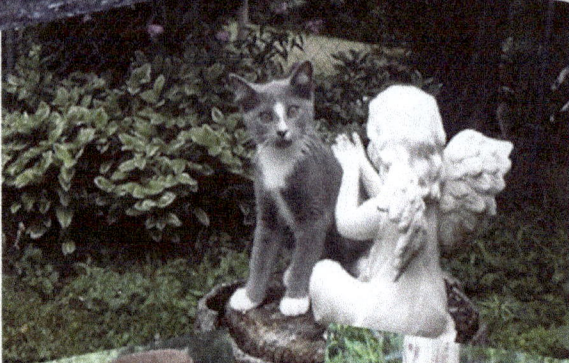
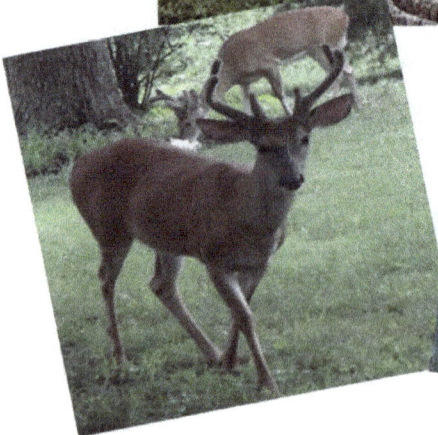
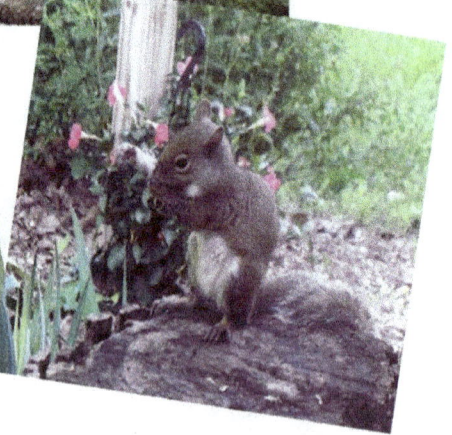

God's Gift of Gentleness

"Let your gentleness be evident to all. The Lord is near."
Philippians 4:5 (NIV)

Gentleness is truly a gift from God. A gentle spirit means that we give up the right to judge what is best for ourselves and others. We stand firm on God's word and allow Him to work in the lives of those around us. Our gentle spirit will show love even in the midst of turmoil.

This does not mean that it is gentle to go easy on people and try to justify actions God calls sin. Paul says in Galatians 6:1: *"If anyone is caught in a trespass, you who are spiritual restore such a one in a spirit of gentleness."*

Gentleness, also translated 'meekness,' does not mean weakness. Rather, it involves humility and thankfulness toward God, and polite, restrained behavior toward others. The opposites of gentleness are anger, a desire for revenge, and self-promotion.

A gentle spirit is not a weak spirit. In the stories that follow, both Ron Miller and Annah Bravata have spiritual strength and fortitude. Annah's gentle spirit is clearly shown in how, as a hospice nurse, she loves and cares for her grandfather.

Ron Miller's gentle spirit shines, while amid illness and sometimes confusion, he continued to paint. His intentions were solely to bring joy to another person as he gave his creations away. His wife did her part as she kept his room stocked with materials he would need.

~Susie

A Passion to Share

"And the peace of God, which transcends all understanding, will guard your hearts and your minds in Christ Jesus."
Philippians 4:7 (NIV)

Finding your passion can seriously change your life. What drives you? What keeps you going when life throws you a curve?

Russell and I developed some great friendships in our community and in the churches where we served for over 20 years. Now that Russell has gone on to glory, I continue to be amazed at what I continue to learn about those God allowed us to serve with.

Russell and I were invited to Ron and Diana Miller's home after church one Sunday to view some beautiful paintings. Of course, we were also there to enjoy a delicious home-cooked meal, complete with a carry-out bag for later!

Through the years, we watched as Brother Ron had to give up his work, much of his driving, and many of his outside activities. Often his memory failed him. And yet, we watched him stay at peace with himself and the world around him. At times, I personally questioned how he could lose so much and yet be such a positive influence on others.

His wife explained, concerning his paintings, that she was continually on the lookout for anything large enough to put a brush to. Pictured are a few of his paintings on old saws that adorn the outside of their home.

Inside, Ron proudly showed us his very own "man cave," well-equipped with an assortment of brushes, trowels, paints, etc. Their walls were a virtual art gallery, displaying beautiful paintings of every size and subject.

Since each visitor was encouraged to choose a painting to take home, we each chose one which he readily autographed for us. He also allowed me to snap photos from his sketchbook in case I might need one for a writing project.

Until that visit, we were unaware of his deep passion for painting. He could go into his "man cave" and create to his heart's content. Just him and his Heavenly Father communing for hours as he worked. He was at peace with His Lord and with himself. He spread joy with his endearing smile and thoughtful words.

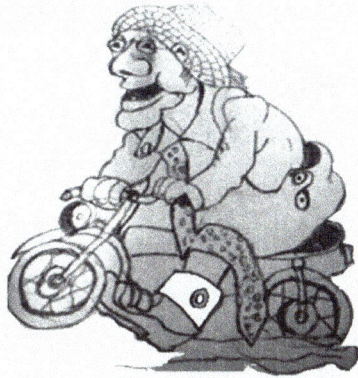

I ask you... Do you know what your passion is? What is it that fulfills the God-given urges inside you? What brings you peace in the midst of your storms?

What is it that you really would like to do if you had the time? I suggest you make the time ... just a little now and then and stir up that passion. It will bring a smile to your heart and spread out into a hungry world.

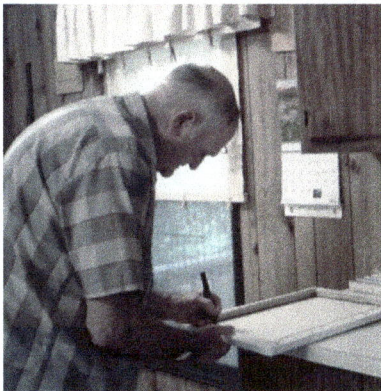

~ Ron Miller's Story as told by Susie Kinslow Adams

High Noon – Sunday

*"Each of you should use whatever gift you have received to serve
others, as faithful stewards of God's grace in its various forms."*
1 Peter 4:10 (NIV)

My mother had a stroke in August 1986. Ron and I visited
her in the hospital. Before we left to go home, Ron asked Mother
if he could borrow one of her "Get Well" cards. I imagine she was
curious about why, but she readily agreed.

In November of 2020, he was unable to go shopping for my
birthday present, so Ron set out to paint the pair of flowers on
Mother's "Get Well" card! I see them each day on my living room
wall... a very sweet memory.

Ron Miller was a quiet man who always needed to keep busy.

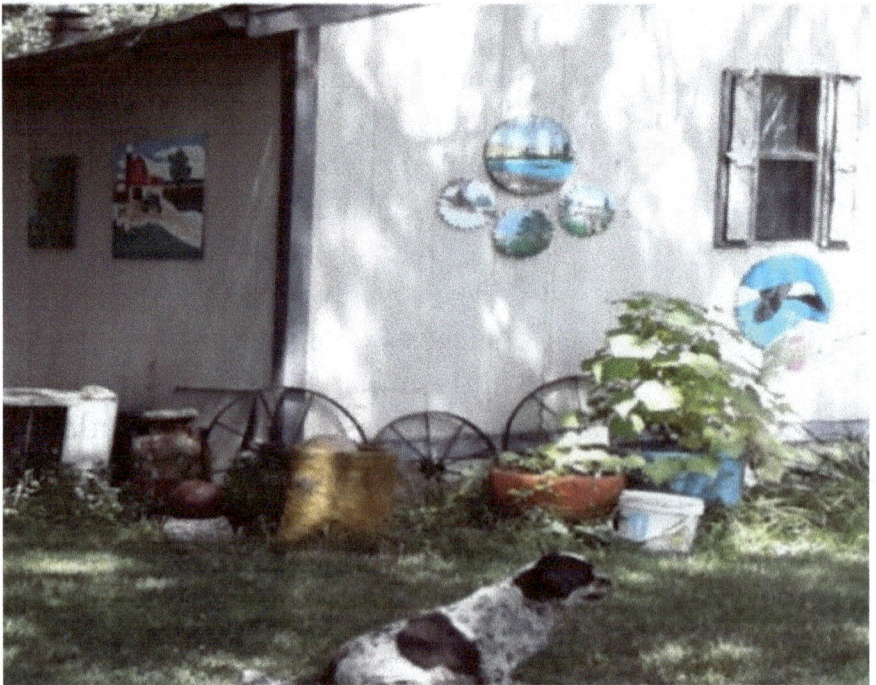

He liked woodworking and made hundreds of fishing lures. He also kept busy painting on hundreds of canvas pieces of various sizes as well as objects - such as glass, wood, and even metal. (It was fun for me to keep an eye out for anything different he could paint on.) When anyone came to visit, they were always invited to choose a canvas from his art gallery wall to take home with them.

When his cancer was diagnosed in July 2021, he underwent surgery. After his hospital stay followed by nursing home care, he came home in September 2021. He spent time watching lots of western movies, which I made sure he had plenty of. Plus, he had his laptop.

Even though Ron was a quiet person, my house is much quieter now. I find things to do to keep myself occupied. But there is no one to talk to or to discuss my problems with. I must make decisions by myself concerning the car, the home, and health issues. I miss him.

The last heartbreaking comment he made to me was, *"I'm glad it's me in this hospital bed- I couldn't do it if you were in my place."*

I will always remember the last breath he took at "High Noon" on Sunday, August 14, 2022.

~Diana M. Miller

I'm Your Nurse, Grandpa

"For if we believe that Jesus died and rose from the dead, so also God will bring with Him those who have fallen asleep through Jesus."
1 Thessalonians 4:14 (NASB)

I walked into your home like every other time before, but this time I knew it would be different. I walked into your home not just as your granddaughter but as your nurse. I left my shoes at the door as always, but today I put on my nurse's hat - I knew this time it would be different.

Yes, I knew today would be the last day I would talk to you here on this earth. I walked into your room to see your eyes closed and you talking away. Although I could not make out the words, you had such a smile on your face. I knelt by your bedside and held your hand for a few minutes, so you knew I was there. Your eyes opened slightly, and you had the most peaceful look about you.

I knew it would be difficult for you to respond to me, as I know how the terminal disease had drained all your energy, but I tried anyway. I said, "Grandpa, are you seeing them yet... your welcoming committee? Did you see Grandma?" You smiled again, paused for quite some time (I know... to get out clear words takes so much effort). Then, in a shallow, low voice, you said, "Yes, yes." My heart felt light, and shivers made the hair on my arms stand up. I said, "Was Uncle John there too?" You paused again for a length of time, then uttered the word, "Yes." I saw joy reflected in your face. I kissed your forehead and said, "You see, Grandpa, there is no fear in death, you're going to the place that was intended for you - a place of unimaginable joy and love - no more fear, no more anxiety, no more doubt, no more disease or pain."

People always speak about how we enter this world; everyone knows the stories, but what to expect in death— no one talks about that. It makes us uncomfortable. Death is just as ordinary as life; it matters. As we labor to be born, we labor in death. Death is a deliverance into the place God has prepared for us. Our earthly body fades, fails, and withers, but our souls long to be reunited with Him.

As a hospice nurse, I share with my patients and their families what the last days may look like and what to expect. It is in those transitional moments I want to share the light and hope; it is in those moments you see life after death. People always say to me, isn't being a hospice nurse difficult? You must always be sad.

But being a hospice nurse is a great honor. It has given me hope beyond the grave; for it is not death we should fear but the absence of God in our hearts and lives. I have less fear of death now than I ever did. I get to witness people being welcomed home. It is their faith, their stories, their interactions with the world beyond, that tells of a greater purpose than this earthly life has ever held. Faith and hope are divine... God's gift to us so we can see beyond our earthly selves.

~Annah Bravata

An Encouraging Word

"For our light and momentary troubles
are achieving for us
an eternal glory
that far outweighs them all."

2 Corinthians 4:17 (NIV)

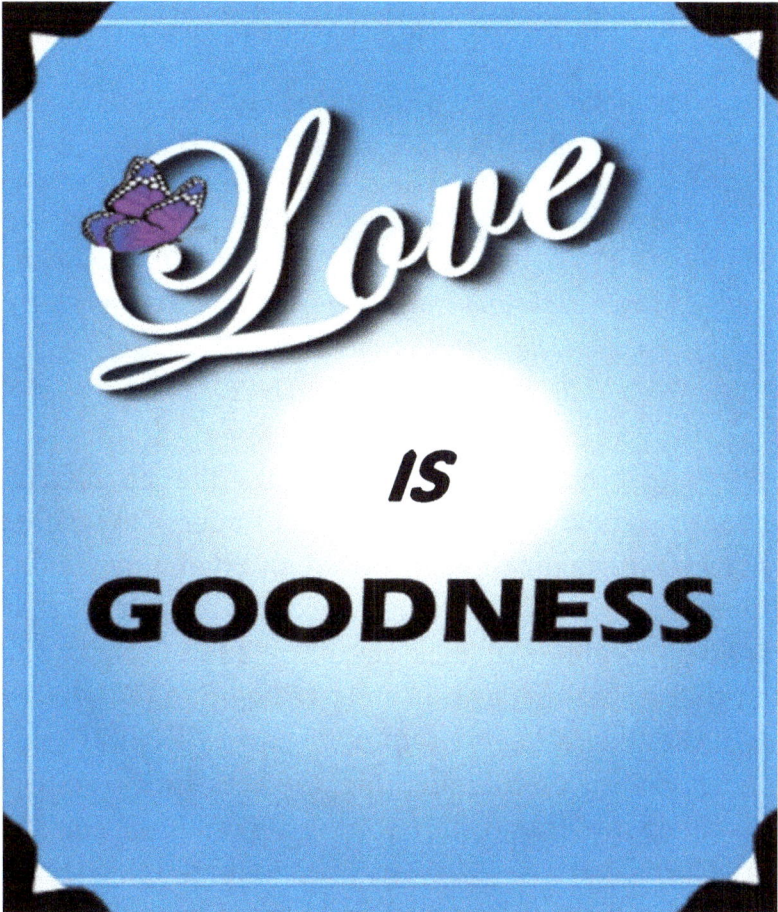

Love

IS

GOODNESS

The Goodness of the Lord

"Therefore, as we have opportunity, let us do good to all people, especially to those who belong to the family of believers."
Galatians 6:10 (NIV)

"I remain confident of this: I will see the goodness of the Lord in the land of the living." Psalm 27:13 (NIV)

"Neither do people light a lamp and put it under a bowl. Instead they put it on its stand, and it gives light to everyone in the house. In the same way, let your light shine before others, that they may see your good deeds and glorify your Father in heaven."
Matthew 5:15-16 (NIV)

It was one of those "God Appointments" that enabled me to know about this next story. On this day, I lingered long after lunch at my favorite pizza place. Although I had much to do before heading home, I could not leave. There was a peace in my heart knowing God was up to something – I felt I must wait to see what that something was. (You have heard of the verse in Isaiah 40:31 that says, *"...wait upon the Lord."* Right?)

Indeed, He was up to something. My long-time friend, Joann Adams, walked into that restaurant for the first time since her husband, Curtis, had passed away. I remembered the pain of all those firsts after Russell had died and invited her to join me until her friends arrived.

When her friends arrived, they joined us. We continued sharing good memories of Curtis and Joann for an hour or more. She needed that time to reminisce. The truth be told, so did I.

As she recounted the story of Curtis' final car ride, her countenance glowed with love and peace. I'm thankful for that meeting. (I might say, *"...my strength was renewed."*) I am thankful for his daughter sharing her story and pictures. I am thankful for and look forward to the grand reunion that awaits all of God's children!

Music provides added dimension to our daily lives. Bart Millard's song, "I Can Only Imagine", has brought special strength to many as we have sought to express our love to the One who loves and forgives us every day of our lives. God speaks to us not only through his word and music but by many different medians. He speaks to us through His Holy Spirit in ways we do not expect. I am thinking we need to start EXPECTING to hear from Him each day.

What do YOU think?

~Susie

Dad's Dream Come True

"Take delight in the Lord, and he will give you the desires of your heart." Psalm 37:4 (NIV)

The Story of Curtis Adams' Final Ride

Last Friday

2:00 pm - Comes home in ambulance and on hospice.

6:00 pm - Goes on a ride that made him smile for days...

- Bigger than he had in years.
- Even got to burn a little rubber.
- I will cherish that moment forever.

I was against the car ride that day. He came home in an ambulance on hospice less than two hours earlier.

The Camaro being there was my husband's idea. Dad had been joking (hard to believe, right?) with Matt about taking our Camaro as collateral for a trailer he was selling us. I didn't expect Dad to say he wanted to go for a ride. None of us did.

I was the only one voicing my concern. However, Dad was adamant; I was vetoed, and I am so thankful that I was. That real, authentic, huge smile on his face was something to see. It had been a very long time since he smiled like that.

That was on a Friday; he continued to smile and tell everyone who came to see or call him about his ride in the hot rod... until Monday evening.

I worked on Monday and stopped at Walmart to pick up a photo book and some more pictures of the car ride. When I got to the house about 6:30 pm he was asleep, but he never fully woke up - awake and coherent. He had been awake and talking up until 15 minutes or so before I got there. Then he passed on Thursday.

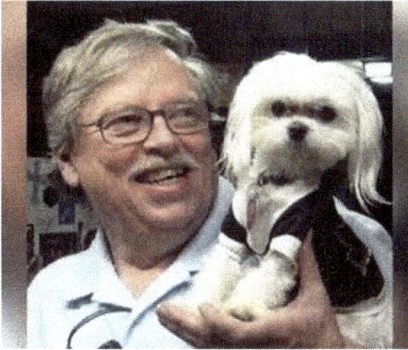

I will never forget that ride or that smile. l miss Dad so much! But it helps to know he's no longer in pain, he can see; and I will see him again someday. When that day comes, "I Can Only Imagine" we'll both be smiling even bigger than the day he got to ride in the hot rod.

~ Curtis Adams as told by daughter, Alma Lindsay

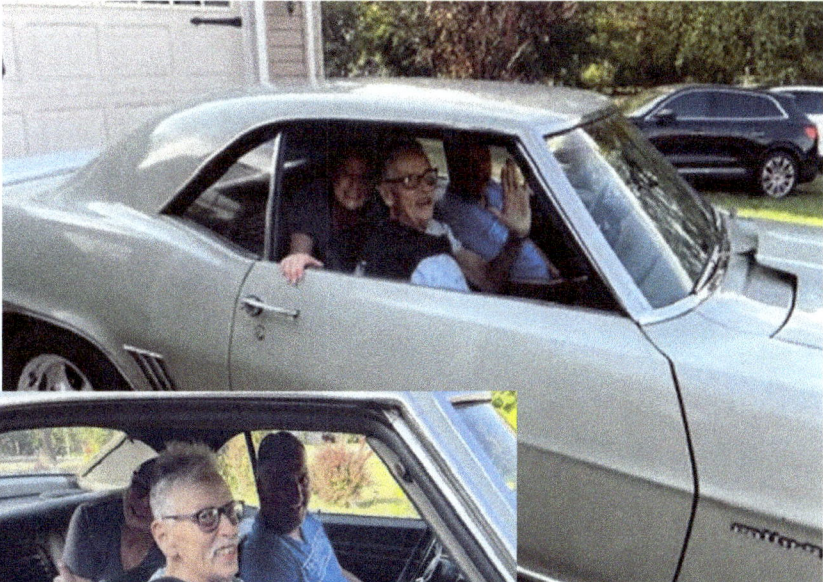

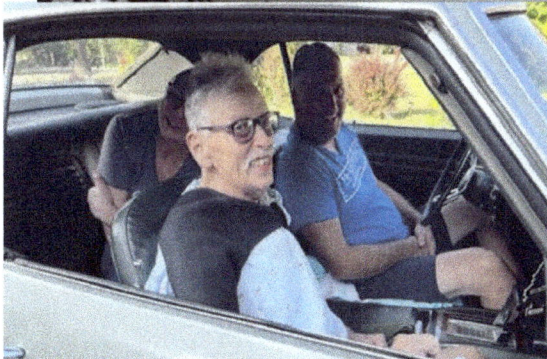

This was a hard time for the Adams family. The impending loss would be huge...and permanent. Yet, in their despair, they chose to make happy memories of their final hours with Dad and Grandpa filled with laughter and joy. This was possible because they knew a reunion in heaven awaits.

~Susie

CHOICES

Even up to our last breath, life is filled with choices.
It's up to us what we choose.

To Remember Me

At a certain moment, a doctor will determine

~that my brain has ceased to function and that, for all intents and purposes, my life has stopped. When that happens, do not attempt to instill artificial life into my body by the use of a machine, and don't call this my deathbed. Let this be called the Bed of Life, and let my body be taken from it to help others lead fuller lives.

~Give my sight *to the man who has never seen a sunrise, a baby's face or love in the eyes of a woman.*

~Give my heart *to a person whose own heart has caused nothing but endless days of pain.*

~Give my blood *to the teenager who was pulled from the wreckage of his car, so that he might live to see his grandchildren play.*

~Give my kidneys *to one who depends on a machine to exist.*

~Take my bones, every muscle, every fiber and nerve in my body and find a way to make a crippled child walk.

~Explore every corner of my brain. Take my cells, *if necessary, and let them grow so that someday a speechless boy will shout at the crack of a bat and a deaf girl will hear the sound of rain against her window.*

~Burn what is left of me and scatter the ashes to the wind to help the flowers grow.

If you must bury something, let it be my faults, my weaknesses and all prejudice against my fellow man.

If by chance you wish to remember me, *do it with a kind deed or a word to someone who needs you. If you do all I have asked, I will live forever.*

~ Robert N. Test

An Encouraging Word

**"There is a time
for everything,
and a season
for every activity
under the heavens:"**

Ecclesiastes 3:1 (NIV)

Love

IS

A

JOURNEY

Together We Journey

"Even though I walk through the darkest valley, I will fear no evil, for you are with me; your rod and your staff, they comfort me."
Psalm 23:4 (NIV)

Have you thought about your journey? Do you sometimes feel you are on a path you do not want to follow? Do you question the hardships of life? I found the definition of journey refreshing as I pondered Mark and Jeanne's journey.

JOURNEY:
~an act or instance of traveling from one place to another.

If we are to look at life as a journey, then by definition, it will have a beginning and an ending. People who do not know Jesus will face their inevitable difficult journeys in fear and trembling. It is easy to be weighed down by the cares of this world when you cannot see your journey's end.

Reading Mark and Jeanne's stories, I believe they knew where each journey would lead. Jeanne had lost parents and in-laws, a sister, a husband, a child, and now her health. And yet she could rejoice with her sisters as they prompted her to sing and focus on Jesus. What amazing joy filled her heart!

An author's confession here: when a friend suggested I ask her brother-in-law for a story, I failed to tell her there was a word limit. When the story came, I was first caught up in the overwhelming details of a trial-filled life. What a powerful testimony of God's grace the two of them shared.

As I considered it for the book, my countenance fell. It was almost three times too long to be included, and I could not figure how to take out over half of it without ruining the story.

While pondering the situation, God arranged it so that I could meet this tall, slim fellow named Mark from Iowa. (Dear reader, I live in the Missouri Ozarks ... only God!) I wish you could have seen his expression as he talked with me about his beautiful "green-eyed lady." Our conversation lingered long as he spoke of God's mercy and healing through it all.

Instead of confessing to him that I couldn't use his story in this book, I asked him to send me pictures. This was one of those times I had to journey into the desert knowing God would provide as I followed Him.

My manuscript has been "almost" finished for some time. However, God gave me no peace until my prayer partners began to pray. There is a purpose for Mark's story; hearts to be mended, lives to be encouraged.

~Susie

Mark's Story

"Finally, brothers and sisters, whatever is true, whatever is noble, whatever is right, whatever is pure, whatever is lovely, whatever is admirable—if anything is excellent or praiseworthy — think about such things." Philippians 4:8 (NIV)

As I write this, it is five months to the day of my beautiful green-eyed lady's death: February 2, 2025. My hope in writing these two stories is that you will clearly see God's hand in all the ups and downs of our forty-two years of marriage.

I have had many careers in my life: I have been a soldier, a member of a consulting engineering company (working as a draftsman, land surveyor field crew, and project inspector), a police officer for six years and finally, for the last nearly thirty years a Registered Nurse, specializing in Emergency Room and Critical Care nursing. Jeanne has been a huge part of these occupations with the exception of soldier. On second glance, my hawkish beliefs and patriotism were tempered by the U.S. Army and became a touchstone in our lives. Her unshakable Faith in Christ anchored me, allowing us to become very involved in our church.

Death has been a frequent visitor. Many milestone events in our life together have been marked by a traumatic event. Jeanne and I met after her first husband died of a massive heart attack at the age of 38. I returned home in the summer of 1978 after my enlistment in the U.S. Army. Jeanne, her husband Richard, and daughters Tricia (11) and Kathryn (7) lived across the street.

My job with the engineering company took me out of town for much of the winter. But as God would have it, when I was home, it seemed as if it snowed every Sunday night. I would shovel Jeanne's walk and driveway at 4:30 a.m., showing a bit of kindness to a family tragically touched by death. One morning, she caught me shoveling! As this petite lady introduced herself, I was captured by the loveliest green eyes I'd ever seen.

As spring turned to summer, I mowed their lawn. She invited me for taco supper with her and the girls! I reciprocated by taking them to a local carnival downtown, complete with rides, including a Ferris wheel and a small roller coaster. Jeanne didn't go on the rides, but her girls rode everything until they got sick.

I soon realized that we were falling in love: Sadly, our dance with Death started soon after. Richard's father died suddenly the next year. Jeanne was still very much involved in his side of the family: Her former mother-in-law was a formidable woman even more petite than Jeanne. A beloved aunt and uncle of Richard's figured very prominently in the girls' lives.

After much discussion with Jeanne and the girls, I asked her to marry me, and on November 27, 1981, we were married. Her daughter, Kathryn, always called it her wedding! And it seemed to me as if I had married not one woman... but three!

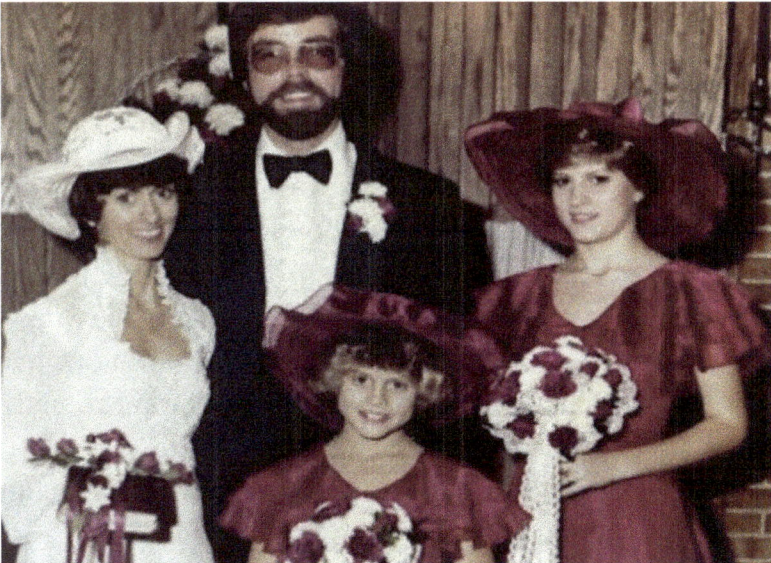

I took a Civil Service Exam in Charles City not realizing it was specific for a job as a police officer. During my time as a cop, both girls graduated from high school and began college. Tricia married her high school sweetheart and moved to a suburb of St. Louis. I left the police department and went back to work for the engineering company.

Spring 1991 the engineering company closed the Charles City office. I had been an ambulance driver for a time and was interested in medicine. With Jeanne's encouragement, I went to school for a nursing degree. For the next two years, I worked as a Nurses' Aide in two care centers every weekend plus two evenings a week.

Death visited twice again during my time in school. Jeanne's mother succumbed to a mysterious ailment. Then not too long after that, Richard's mother, Beatrice, had a minor heart attack and came to live with us to rest and recuperate. After a second heart attack, she lived long enough for both sides of the family to gather and say goodbye. One of my bittersweet memories is of our daughter, Kathryn, curled up alongside her grandmother as she lay dying.

I graduated in the Spring of 1994; the Nursing Board exams were set for July 11, 1994, in Des Moines, Iowa. Jeanne and I went the day before to relax before exams. Jeanne called the girls to let them know our plans. Kathryn was going to a popular lake and park for the afternoon with her boyfriend and other recent graduates. Tricia and her husband were busy with their lives in St. Louis. No one else knew exactly where we were staying.

This is when death became a very real specter in our lives. After a very nice meal, we retired to our small motel room to relax. At 5:30 a.m. the next morning, a Polk County Deputy Sheriff knocked on our door. I looked past him, thinking our car had been hit. "Good morning, officer. What's going on?"

"Are you the Narvesons, and are you the parents of Kathryn Heller?" My blood went cold. I had delivered this message several times to families; I knew what was next.

He said, "I'm sorry, Sir. There's been an accident..."

I gathered Jeanne up in my arms, pulling a robe around her, "Something's happened."

Stone-faced, he delivered the worst news a parent could ever receive: "Your daughter was involved in a car accident about 4:30 p.m. yesterday afternoon, apparently heading to Ames from Big Creek. The driver of the car missed a stop sign on the county road, entered the intersection at highway speed, and was struck on the passenger side door by a pickup going north. Of the four people in the car, only the driver survived."

Jeanne and I collapsed on the bed while the deputy left paperwork as to where Kathryn had been taken. As we later found out, Kathryn's boyfriend had been driving her car at the time. He was in the hospital with a severe head injury; the other two boys and Kathryn had been killed.

It had taken all night to find us because friends and family only knew we were in Des Moines... but not where we were lodging. They had been calling every motel and hotel in the Des Moines metro area all night trying to find us.

Our world unraveled as we called friends and family. The next weeks were a blur of funeral arrangements, the clans gathering, and the awful truth of never again seeing our vivacious and caring young lady. Now, we were trying to adjust to life without her.

Passing my boards three months later, I began working full-time at one of the nursing homes where I had worked while going to school. We moved several times; always wanting to be close to our family when possible.

Death has a way of destroying things. I remember well a call from my mother. "Your Dad has had a heart attack. It doesn't look good." They didn't have much hope yet agreed to keep him sedated and ventilated for three days. *He was admitted to the very floor where I was to start the next week.* (Only God can orchestrate these events as we learn to follow His guidance.)

My last duty to my father was to shave him before he was transferred to the hospital in Charles City under hospice care.

Jeanne and I were at his bedside when I told my exhausted family to go home and get some rest. We sat there lost in our thoughts for about two hours when, just like that, he stopped breathing. I believe my father waited until his family had gone home before he took his final journey. He knew Jeanne and I had the strength to cope.

It was around this time that Jeanne was diagnosed with Myotonic Dystrophy, a form of Muscular Dystrophy that occurs later in life. This was what had probably killed Jeanne's mother. It is a gradual wasting of muscles, starting with fine muscle control. She began to lose strength in her hands, and her balance was affected.

Jeanne retired in about 2006, and I took a position in the ER. Later, in 2013, I worked in another ER known for gangs and gang violence on the East Side of Waterloo; I was in my element. After four years there, Jeanne and I decided to return to Mercy North Iowa in Mason City. I applied, and to my surprise, the current director of CCU was a friend from my time in that ER. I said, "Can I come back?" She said, "Absolutely!" and my interview consisted of the two of us trading "war stories."

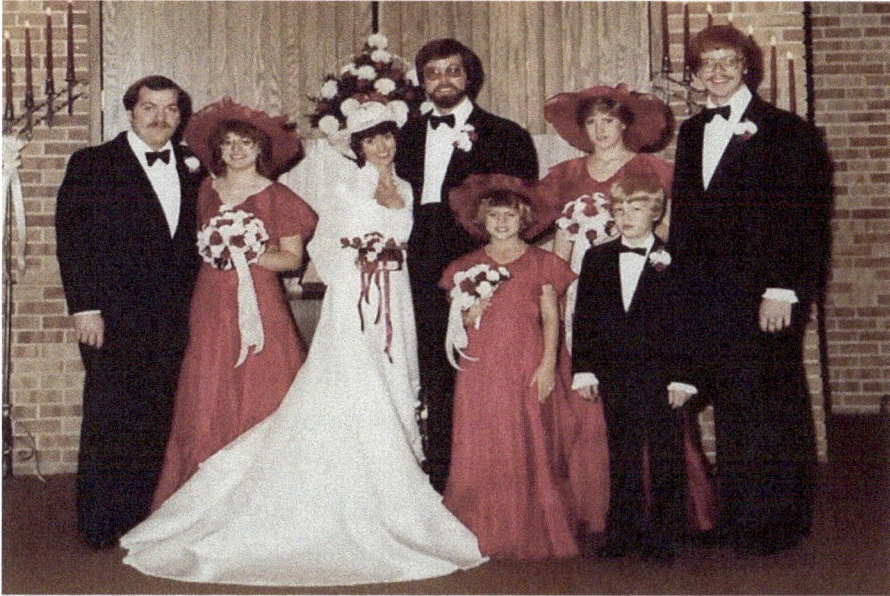

So, this brings me to the final phase of my career and ultimately, Jeanne's life and legacy. From August of 2017, I was "home" at Mercy in Mason City. Jeanne had begun to show definite signs of Myotonic Dystrophy (DM) causing more problems with her health. We even removed our back doorsteps and installed a custom half-riser set of steps that doubled the number of steps but cut the height of each step in half, such that Jeanne only had to barely lift her foot, and she was on the next step.

My life from army days forward has been one of facing illnesses, death, tragedies, and losses head-on. What I could not know is that my greatest challenge and loss was just beginning to reveal itself.

~ Mark Narveson

Green-Eyed Lady

"And Adam said, This is now bone of my bones, and flesh of my flesh: she shall be called Woman, because she was taken out of Man. Therefore shall a man leave his father and his mother, and shall cleave unto his wife: and they shall be one flesh." Genesis 2:23-24 (KJV)

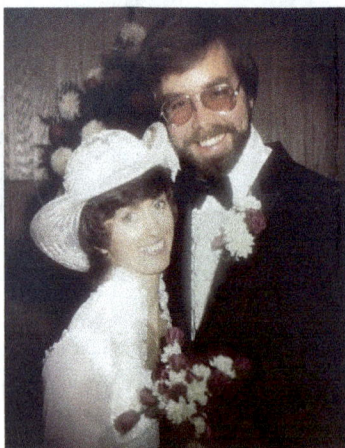

When my beautiful green-eyed lady died, I did not simply lose another person in my life; I lost a part of me. God was not using a metaphor when He said, "they shall be one flesh." There is a hole in my heart that no one can fill. However, by God's grace, I can be thankful for the years we were given, and I can trust His plan for my future.

I was Jeanne's primary caregiver during the last eleven months of her life. I treasure those times; I feel honored to have had the opportunity to be with her as she prepared for her final journey Home.

For much of our life together, especially upon returning to North Iowa and our lovely Craftsman home, Jeanne would go on "Sisters Weekends" with her sisters, Ruth, Evelyn, and Marilyn; usually meeting in Kansas City or St. Louis. Gradually, as age and health issues began to affect each of us, I was granted the title of "Honorary Sister" and allowed to participate in the weekend getaways. In addition to Jeanne's health issues, Marilyn succumbed to a severe lung condition and Evelyn had a reaction to Levaquin which affected her walking for a time. All husbands were invited, but the others declined. Jeanne and I would drive to a motel near Kansas City International Airport. Evie would drive up from Fair Play, Missouri. Ruth would fly in from Nashville, Tennessee. I was the chauffeur and heavy lifter. There were several theaters, stores, and restaurants nearby. Strangely enough, I have always loved to shop, so I was a good fit. (God takes care of the details!)

As 2023 arrived, our "Sisters Weekends" included celebrating surviving the COVID Pandemic. Jeanne's health began to decline rapidly that year.

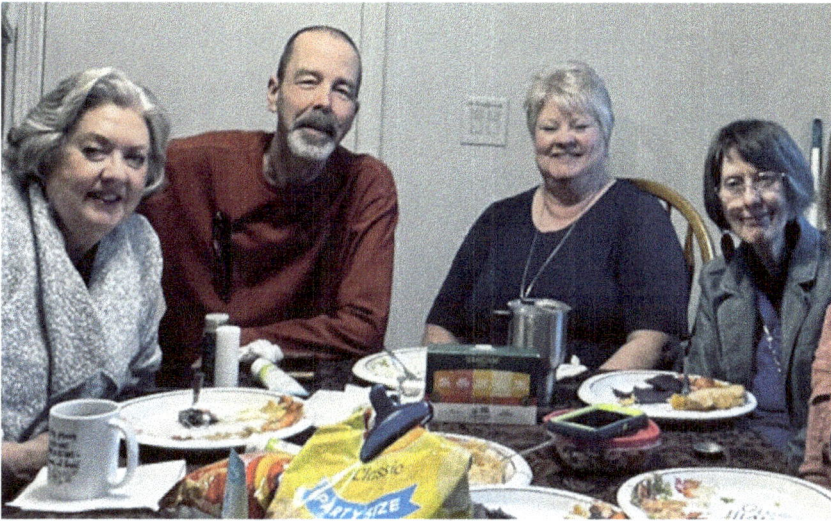

Three amazing ladies: our daughter Tricia and Jeanne's sisters, Ruth and Evie, took turns taking care of Jeanne, allowing me to continue work. As her health slowly declined, she kept her spirits up. Evie and Ruth made "flash cards" of her favorite Bible verses and hung large posters of inspirational sayings where she could easily see them. In her weakest moments, she would read them and smile.

On Wednesday, August 23rd, 2023, I had a meeting and did a little shopping after it was over. When I got home, Jeanne was uncharacteristically angry at me. She began walking around in circles in the dining room. When I asked where she was going, she replied, "I need the bathroom!" I directed her toward the bathroom, but she headed into the kitchen. "Now, where are you going?" I asked. She snapped, "To the bathroom!"

I feel I should have recognized her behavior as symptoms of a deeper issue. I had given her flash cards, and they were resting on her left leg. When she asked where her cards were, I said they were on her left leg. She began to pat her right leg saying she didn't see them. I said, "Your OTHER left." Which really made her angry.

It finally began to dawn on me what was happening: "Can you see the cards on your left leg?" I asked. "No," she replied. I pointed to the word at the top of the poster: It was SALVATION. "What is this word?" When she replied "ON", I realized that she was having Left Vision Field Loss! She was having a stroke! All my training at stroke detection was right out the window.

Calling 911 would take too long. I picked Jeanne up, carried her to the car and raced to the ER. Recognizing the nurse at the Triage desk, I said, "She's having a stroke, and we're out of the window!" She was whisked away to have a CT scan. I parked the car and hurried back in. I could hear hushed conversations as each team member arrived outside her door. The gist was mostly, "It's Mark's wife..." "Does he know....?" "He was in the control room; he knows."

Eventually, Jeanne was admitted to Critical Care (MY floor), just outside the main nurses' station, and treated like a queen by my "work family". Visits from family, our pastor, church friends, and others from the past helped her settle down.

When the day of surgery arrived, we accompanied her down to the Surgery area and settled in the Waiting Room. All too soon, the Neurosurgeon came in with a grim look on his face. He was straightforward in explaining the complications he had faced. "She came through what surgery we could do and is in Recovery. She'll be in her room soon. We'll keep her lightly sedated while she recovers." When pressed about follow-up treatment, he stated, "There is radiation and chemotherapy, but these kinds of tumors don't respond well to chemo." Then, the bombshell: "She has a six-to-twelve-month life expectancy."

So, back in her room in Critical Care, Jeanne began to awaken. Wonder of wonders, she was very much like her prior self: Witty, charming, and much more concerned for those around her rather than herself. A few days later, she was transferred to the Skilled Nursing Unit, and at this place, she flourished: She was walking again (with a walker) and her appetite had returned! August 23rd she weighed about 95 lbs.; now she weighed about 110 lbs.

Homecoming was set for the end of September 2023. She was comfortable back on her couch, still able to get around. With frequent stays from Tricia, Ruth, and Evie, I could still manage to work a little. The Hospice staff people were terrific: There was a young lady who was part of music therapy who would come with a guitar to play and sing for us. On the days that Tricia or Evie were here, they would play piano, and we would have a singalong. Very often, Jeanne would fall asleep singing with the most peaceful smile on her face.

As time went on and 2023 became 2024, she gradually grew weaker. I went to work on the morning of June 6, 2024 (the 80th anniversary of D-Day) and approached my boss, Emily, in her office. "I don't think I can continue here anymore. Jeanne is requiring more care, and I want to be with her until...."

Returning home, I felt truly released from my responsibility to the hospital and I could care for Jeanne in earnest. It was timely as Jeanne took a very decided downturn from the second week in June. At about 6:30 on the morning of July 2nd, for some reason, I got up and went out to check on her. She was very still. Her body was still warm. I think that she passed just as I got to her bedside. Ruth and Evie had stayed longer than usual, due to the way Jeanne had deteriorated. They were sleeping upstairs. I quickly summoned them and called Tricia, and we had a long period of silence. I don't remember much of those first few minutes. This was not unexpected, but it was unexpectedly final.

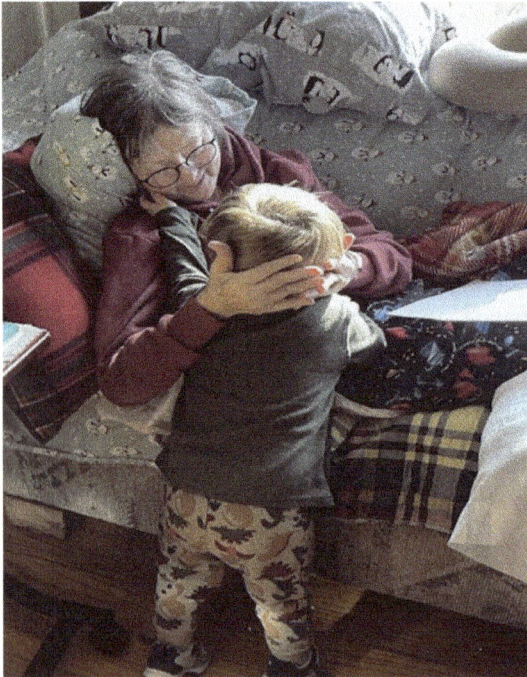

After our daughter, Kathryn, had died years before, we had purchased two burial plots just below and to the right of Kathryn's plot. Jeanne would be buried just kitty-corner to Kathryn's feet. Eventually, I'll be buried on Jeanne's left. Jeanne and I kind of laughed about what people in the future would think as they looked at the graves and all the different names interred there.

When first setting up all the particulars at the funeral home, we made it clear that Jeanne had wanted all of the best "stuff". But over the years, even before her stroke, she had again made it very clear she did NOT want an expensive funeral. In fact, she insisted on "renting" a casket for the funeral, after which, she said, "Then just put me in a pine box." Tricia and I were appalled, but the Funeral Director had an idea: "I may have a solution. We have a medium-duty casket in the back that is a very nice metal. But a few months ago, we were moving another casket, and it fell putting a big dent at the bottom of this one. We can look at it and I'll give it to you for half-price." We all burst out laughing: "A scratch and dent casket!! She'd love that."

AND SO, IT WAS.

In the months that have passed, my health has returned. At the time of the funeral, I weighed 142 lbs. I am 6' 3" and I looked like a scarecrow. In late August, I received an Insulin pump, and my blood sugars have returned largely to normal. By December my weight had climbed to 165 lbs. My "normal" weight is 185 lbs. (which is still a bit thin). My thought processes are much clearer, and I have begun to enjoy retirement. I still have episodes of grief and I swear I can hear her sweet voice occasionally. Usually, it's a very definite, "NO!" When I'm thinking about writing a letter to the editor or something like that. It is good to know she is still watching out for me.

~Mark Narveson

An Encouraging Word

"Peace I leave with you;
my peace I give you.
I do not give to you
as the world gives.
Do not let your hearts be troubled
and do not be afraid."

John 14:27 (NIV)

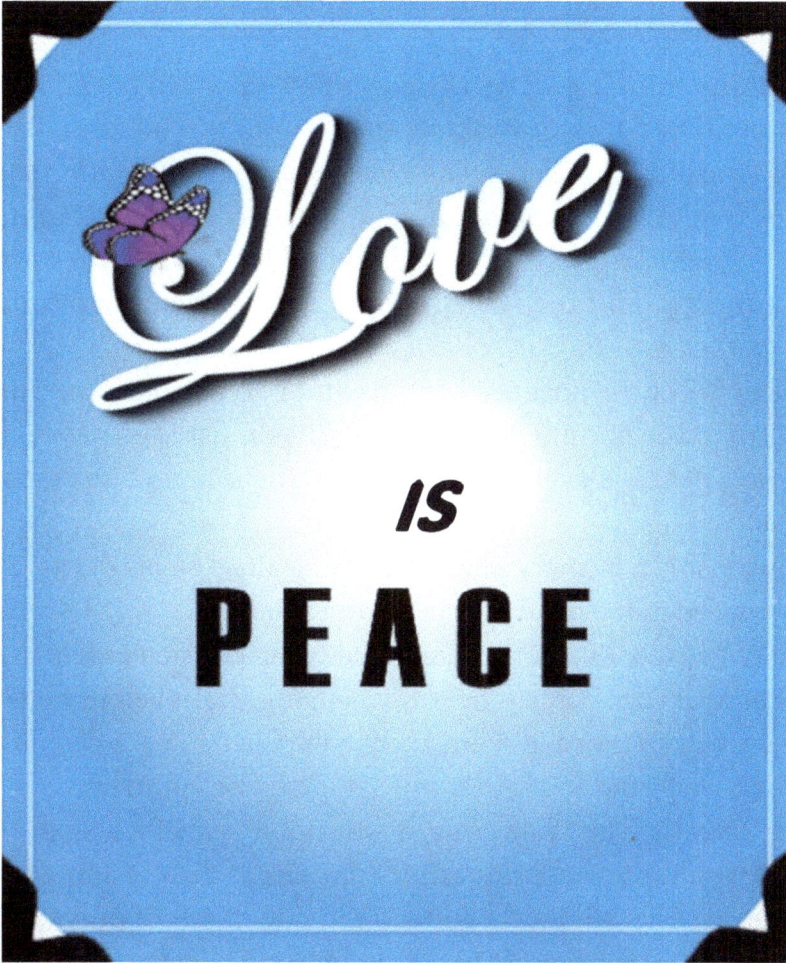

Love

IS

PEACE

God's Perfect Peace

"You will keep him in perfect peace, Whose mind is stayed on You, Because he trusts in You." Isaiah 26:3 (NKJV)

In Philippians 4:6-7, we are admonished not to be anxious about anything but to pray about every situation. I like the J.B. Phillips translation which says, *"Don't worry over anything whatever; tell God every detail of your needs in earnest and thankful prayer, and the peace of God which transcends human understanding, will keep constant guard over your hearts and minds as they rest in Christ Jesus."*

Peace is not the absence of trials and tribulations. We cannot muster up peace of our own accord, but we must seek peace from God. God's peace is everlasting - even in the midst of our most violent storms.

How vividly a memory of my dad sitting alone on his old painter's bench is etched in my mind. It was a warm summer day as Mother and I rushed out the door to go shopping. Daddy's expression caught my eye as I hurried past; perhaps he was hoping for a chat before we left. But we were in a hurry and scurried on to the car.

When we found my father after he had chosen to end his pain the only way he knew how, it was not a peaceful scene. Comfort would come, but not immediately. For quite some time, there was an internal battle going on inside of me. If only... I should have... This was not to be the only such time our family would face these "what ifs" in our lives.

Cindy puts things in perspective when she created a beautiful family photo setting, which included a prominent place for her son's bible to complete their family photo. He is forever in her heart and soon will be in her arms again when all are gathered Home.

Another challenge to making peace with our past is finding peace as we face role reversals. Our parents were the ones we ran to when trials came. Only through God's unfailing love and mercy are we able to realize real peace as we take on the role of parenting our parents.

In *My Mother My Child,* I described how difficult it was to realize Momma wasn't coming back. This person in her shell had no recollection of being my mother and no desire to do so. Rebecca says it well in her story: "The most difficult part of the whole process was in my own heart because the mental process of having to parent your own parent isn't easy."

Dear reader, wherever you are on your journey through this life, I pray you know the peace of God in the midst of your storms.

~Susie

From My Hands to His

"For I am the LORD, your God, who takes hold of your right hand, Who says to you, 'Do not fear, I will help you.'" Isaiah 41:13 (NASB)

My caregiving journey with my mother began in November of 2015 when we moved her from California to Missouri to be near me in her final years. Looking back, I now realize we should have moved her much sooner, but the Lord has His timing and worked it all out for us. We were able to move her into a small house just down the street from us where I cared for her for six short years until she passed from this world into the next.

Mom had always said I lived with my head in the clouds and I am sure she was correct; because even though I was my mother's only biological child, the concept of elder care had never even crossed my mind... that is until I was hit in the face with it just a year or two before she came to be with me.

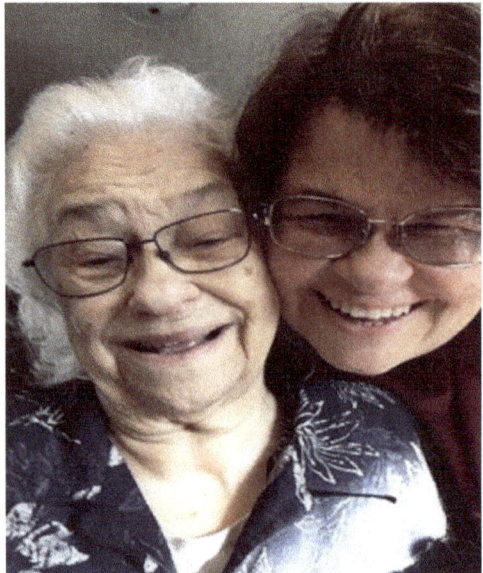

Mom seemed to be doing well living on her own into her mid-eighties, but unbeknownst to me, dementia had set in, and she was rapidly deteriorating mentally. She needed help with virtually everything and was no longer able to drive safely. I was blessed that Mom was an agreeable, happy-go-lucky person and didn't fight me too much as we gradually transferred more and more responsibilities from her hands to mine, driving, bank account, medicines, etc. The most difficult part of the whole process was in my own heart because the mental process of having to parent your own parent isn't easy.

As time progressed, so did her dementia. Do not be fooled—dementia is a heartbreaking foe. Mom forgot much of her past and wondered why family members hadn't contacted her lately. Inexplicably, she remembered my name and that I was her daughter until the very end but only had dim recollections of being married. Dementia may have taken her memories, but it didn't take her joy, nor her faith. She delighted in every sunrise, every blooming flower, and every bird at the bird feeder. She loved to read her Bible and sing the old hymns. It seemed that as dementia destroyed her ties to the world, it opened the portals of heaven, and her faith was what remained, simple but unconquerable.

Mom passed from my hands into His hands on December 24, 2021. It was a privilege to have cared for her in her last years. The caregiving walk with her wasn't easy, but the Lord was with us and blessed us with loving friends and neighbors, without whose help we wouldn't have been able to keep her at home until the end.

~Rebecca D. Howard

God Gathers His Lambs

"See, the Lord God comes with strength, and His power establishes His rule. His reward is with Him, and His gifts accompany Him. He protects His flock like a shepherd; He gathers the lambs in his arms and carries them in the fold of His garment. He gently leads those that are nursing."
Isaiah 40:10-11 (HCSB)

Gatherings around the table have always been an important part of my life. I remember as a child, BIG family dinners on every holiday. As David and I started our own family, those gatherings continued to be very important to us. We would gather at Grandma Dorothy's for our annual Christmas Eve seafood feast and celebration, or at Grandma Lilly's on Christmas Day for ham, mashed potatoes, delicious white gravy, and brown and serve rolls. As our children grew into adulthood and started their own families, the traditions of gathering continued. Our family not only has a deep love for food and gatherings, but a deeper love for each other.

In 2020, our lives drastically changed. Our oldest son, Brian, and his wife had filed for divorce. Brian was able to join our family traditions, but it was unbearable for him without his children. Brian was raised in the church - including VBS and Sunday School (with the famous Margaret Hamlet and Catherine Crump as teachers). At the age of 10, Brian and I made a trip to Lake of the Ozarks, and on the way home, in the backseat of our car, Brian asked Jesus to forgive him of his sins and be His Savior. But, as with many teenagers and young adults, church and Jesus were often replaced with friends and fun. I often talked to Brian about his relationship with Jesus and prayed for him (and all my children) every day.

In late 2021, Brian met an amazing woman who loved Jesus. Kayla and her family were answers to my many prayers. Kayla's dad kept asking Brian to go to church with them. Brian started attending church and re-dedicated his life to the Lord. We had several conversations about his bible readings and the bible studies they were doing. I could see a change in his life and in his heart. I could also see the inward struggles he was experiencing from his ongoing divorce and custody battles. Brian was a very private person and carried so much weight of his struggles alone. On August 2, we lost our son. His struggles became too much for him to bear. Our family would never be the same. There was an aching, gaping hole in our hearts and around that precious dining room table.

I had wanted to do family pictures for some time, but we never captured family photos before his death because we wanted his children in the photos. God's mercy, grace, and comfort have been my constant companion. There are days that I can literally feel God answering the prayers of dear friends helping me to pick up one foot and place it in front of the other. I have poured over scriptures to find peace. I have worshiped when all I could do was take all my emotion and pour it out to Him. I decided that part of my healing would be to get those family photos completed.

Honestly, two days before the scheduled shoot, I was ready to call and cancel. I couldn't think of having family photos without him. I prayed and asked God to help me because I felt it would be an important step not only for my healing but our family's healing. God helped me find a way I could include Brian in our family photo. I went to Brian's Bible that he had given himself on Father's Day 2022; a bookmark was in Isaiah, chapter 40. He had marked verses 10 and 11 where God's word talks about how He gathers His lambs and protects them in the fold of His garment. I am comforted knowing Brian had found peace that God would protect and watch over his kids in his absence. Because he had given His heart to Jesus, I also have peace knowing... he is sheltered in the arms of Jesus. Brian's Bible now rests on the picnic table as we gather for family photos.

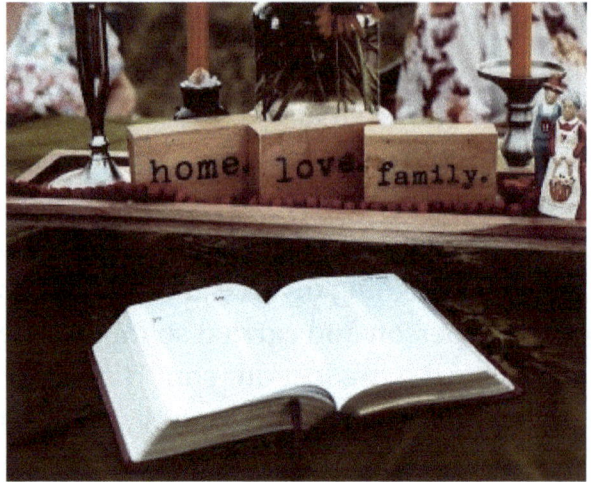

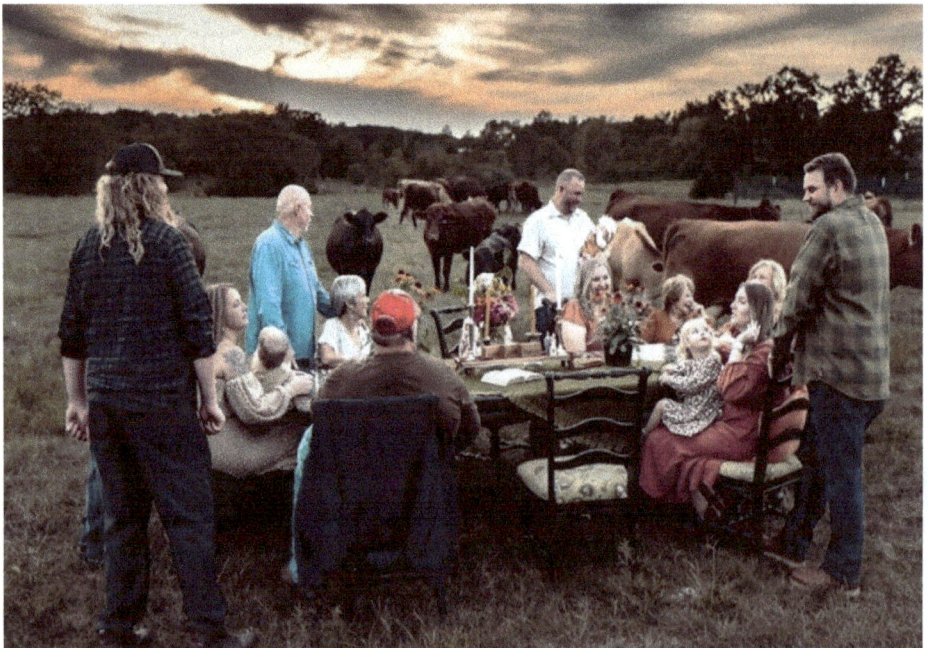

Our pictures reflect God's goodness in our lives. A reflection of our family and its love, strength, and our legacy of the "gatherings". God clearly made His presence known to us through His creation that day by enveloping our family in a sky that speaks of His goodness. Healing came in the form of laughs that speak of our resilience and our love for each other. I look forward to heaven-the GREAT gathering, where we can all be together again. I kind of think there will be a big dining room table filled with all our favorites... enjoying each other and praising our Savior for eternity.

~ Cindi Lockhart

An Encouraging Word

**You make known to me
the path of life;
you will fill me
with joy in your presence,
with eternal pleasures
at your right hand.**

Psalm 16:11 (NIV)

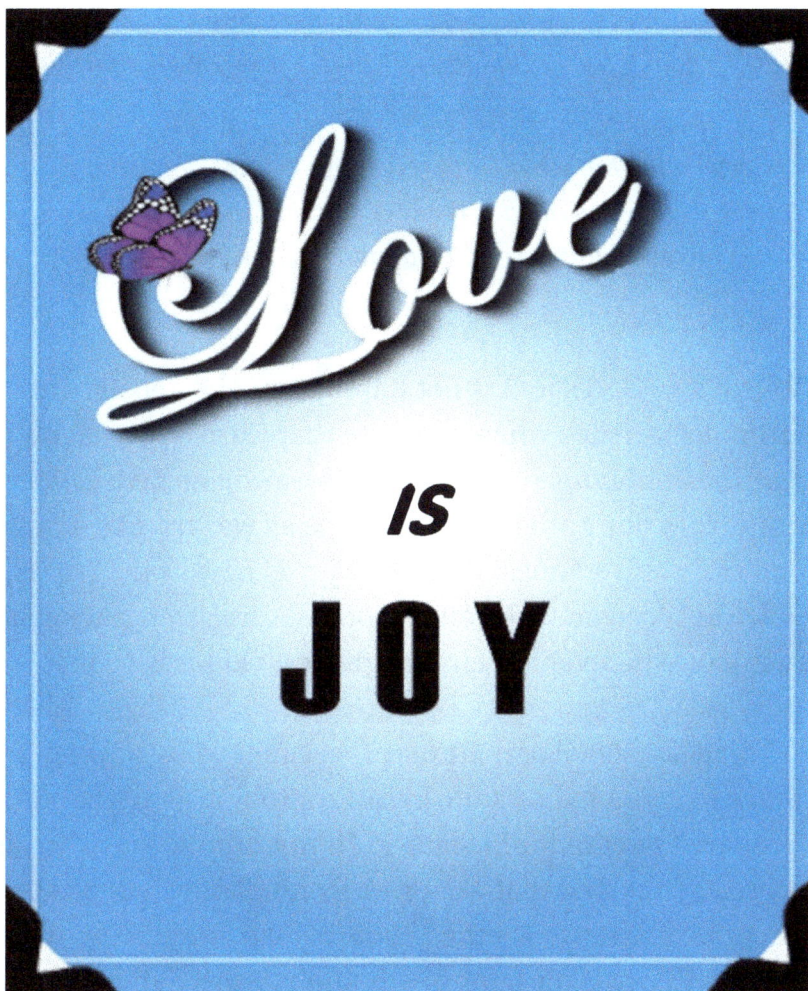

Love

IS

JOY

Understanding God's Joy

"Count it all joy, my brothers, when you meet trials of various kinds, for you know that the testing of your faith produces steadfastness."
James 1:2-3 (ESV)

"Our hearts ache, but we always have joy. We are poor, but we give spiritual riches to others. We own nothing, and yet we have everything." 2 Corinthians 6:10 (NLT)

Biblical joy (God's joy) is not happiness. The apostle Paul spoke from experience when he wrote that Christians can be *"sorrowful, yet always rejoicing;"* (2 Corinthians 6:10 ESV). This word from our Father gives us hope as we strive to ease the suffering of our loved ones. Our inner joy is never taken away. We rejoice as forgiven children of God. We are strengthened as we remember whatever the circumstances, God is with us.

As I read *The Love of a Father*, I was moved by how an experience in a young boy's life became a tool in God's hands as Dave prepared to care for his father. In this simple story, we are encouraged by the fact that not one second of our lives has been wasted. As we learn to turn the good, the bad, and the ugly over to God, He will use it for our growth and maturity and for His glory.

Close your eyes and picture that loving son cradling his father in his arms one last time. Dear reader, if you do not know for sure your Heavenly Father will do that for you, we need to talk.

As you read Annah's poem, *Life Giver*, let the last stanza soak into your being. Close your eyes and feel the joy that comes from knowing - really knowing we have a home awaiting us. Picture your grand reunion with loved ones so dear.

Oh, what JOY!

~Susie

The Love of a Father

"As a father has compassion on his children, so the LORD has compassion on those who fear him." Psalm 103:13 (NIV)

When I was five years old, I jumped with both feet into the bathtub like any five-year-old might do. Within seconds, I realized that I had turned the hot water on but no cold water. I jumped out of the tub to see my skin was burnt with second and third-degree burns. I still have scars on the top of my feet today.

I still remember the next day; my father carried me like a baby in his arms through the building to our doctor. I remember feeling infantile being carried like that. After all, I was five years old, and it was unsettling to be carried like that.

I asked my father the other day if he remembered carrying me to the doctor's office. He smiled and nodded yes. I told him, "Now it's my turn."

I lifted Dad into the hospital bed provided by Hospice today....

Life had come full circle.

* * *

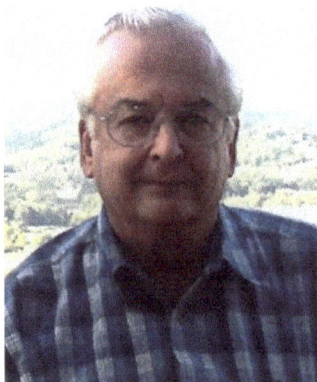

My father went to be with Jesus on Sunday morning; he was originally told that he had three years to live, but instead he lived twelve years after his kidney diagnosis. Dad lived a full life. He was married to Mom for sixty-six years. They met at a church youth group. I believe he was 12 and she was 11 – if I remember that right; so, they were friends for 75 years. (Please remember my mom, Clare, in your prayers. Thank you).

My father's favorite expression I grew up hearing was "If you're going to do something, do it right." I know he influenced me in many ways. I miss him a lot already but look forward to being reunited in heaven someday. I feel blessed and grateful to have been his son, and I will always be thankful for the borrowed time we were allowed to have.

~Dave Kolstedt

Life Giver-The Gift is Life After Death

"But these have been written that you may believe that Jesus is the Christ, the Son of God; and that believing you may have life in His name." John 20:31 (NASB)

Years gone by, this shell running dry
Mortality awaits my soul's certain fate
The unknown, so many questions,
will I meet Him on His heavenly throne?
Is this it… the abyss?
Oh, be still my soul, for it has been foretold
Blood spilt for me, to be free, to gain eternity
Leaving kin and friend, to what end?
Mere mortal, can't you see? Only true life comes through He
He is the Life Giver, the truth seer

You have worked with haste, to find your earthly place
Years of toil, working to build upon this earthly soil
You cling to it, trying to fill the void
Silence the noise, unburden your soul, be a fool no more
For it is not here your kingdom awaits
Feel your bones, how they ache, come claim your heavenly place
For He says, confess to me, come rest in me
I have set aside your place, a realm absent the concerns you face
All that is Divine and Holy

As we labor in birth, we labor in death, it is rebirth, a renewal
Shedding off this earthy skin, entering a realm with Him
Death a portal, it is the open door which leads to more. Trust in Him
He is the Life Giver, the forgiver
He hears your heart,
He sees your tears, wants to relinquish your fears
Let Him take your burden, surrender your fears,
    give him all your years
He has not forgotten you, you He has chosen,
    you He has woven
He knew you from birth, gave you that thirst
Breath of His breath, flesh of His flesh, blood of his blood

Earth is the test, come find your rest
He has awaited you, His beloved
You will be greeted by miles of hearts;
    you did impact-even a small part
No greater love than this, pure Bliss
Erase and embrace this
Let it all go, your life of woe
And on that day
You will hear them sing
Come my child,
    come dance now with your heavenly King

    ~ Annah Bravata

An Encouraging Word

**"Surely your goodness and love
will follow me
all the days of my life,
and I will dwell
in the house of the Lord
forever."**

Psalm 23:6 (NIV)

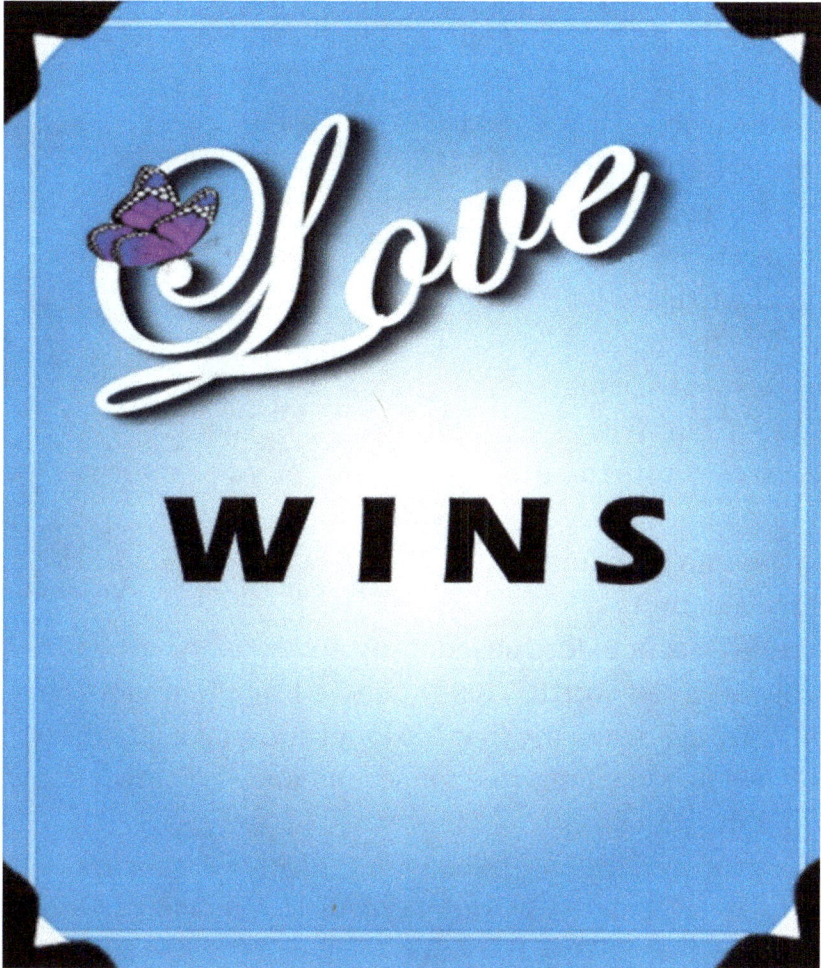

Alone Again

"Trust in the Lord with all your heart, And lean not on your own understanding; In all your ways acknowledge Him, And He shall direct your paths." Proverbs 3:5-6 (NKJV)

My precious Russell celebrates his fourth year in Heaven as this book goes to print. I would like to leave you with a few thoughts about this journey into singleness. Surviving spouses lose more than their loved ones. Lifestyles and schedules undergo a definite change. We seem to lose our identity and sense of confidence, possibly even self-worth. This truth was brought home to me many years ago when my first husband suffered a fatal heart attack. We had been married for seventeen years. I was in my 30's, and he was 44.

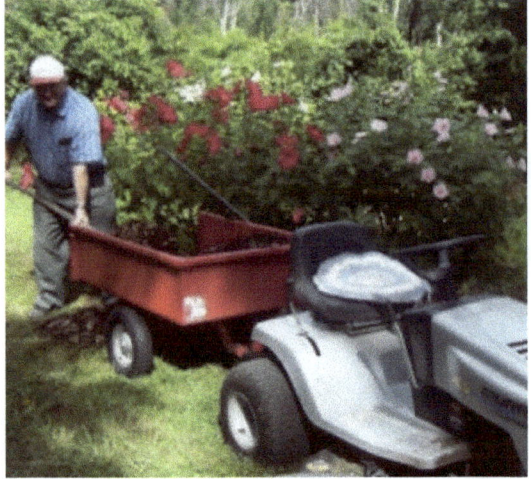

My grocery cart, half-filled with pork chops, sausage, biscuits, sweet rolls, and a variety of snacks, was left abandoned in the aisle. For the first time since Bob's fatal heart attack, I began to realize how much of my life centered around his needs. Those were his favorite foods; I didn't know how to shop for just myself! Paralyzed, I sat in my hot car, tears flowing down my cheeks. I was weary, embarrassed, lonely, and confused.

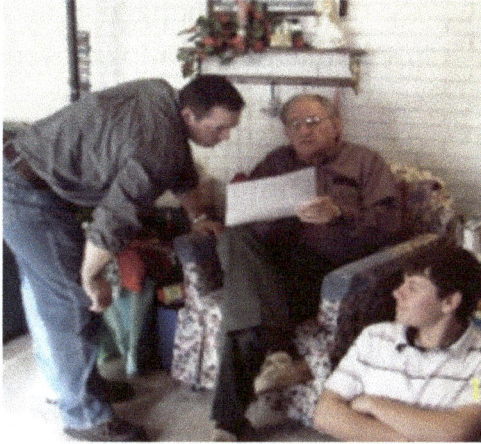

Faith played an important part in my finding my way through those uncharted waters. In 1979, I remarried, and God blessed me with another companion. After forty-plus years, the shadow of widowhood again found my doorstep.

Once again, my daily routines changed. What I cooked for meals and how my spare time was spent were all turned upside down. I had depended solely on my husband to take care of our cars, the furnace, the well, the yard. Now it was up to me to keep things going.

Russell had been serving a group of churches as Director of Missions since the year 2000. On any given Sunday we either were visiting, or he was preaching in one of them. While my membership remains in a church we helped start years ago, I find myself visiting others on special occasions. Many of the kids we saw off to camp in 2000 are now sending their children to camp. I feel like their Granny! God's Family IS FAMILY to me!

My circle of friends didn't change so much, but the things I do with them have changed. Whereas my "hubby" and I did almost everything together, now I must forge ahead as a single person – often feeling like a third wheel. It's not the same without Russell along to help visit with their husbands.

Family relations will change for many widowed people. Not the immediate family so much, but the extended family. His or her family may soon quit calling. It happens - maybe because they think we are too busy, or there may be feelings of uncertainty, such as – "Does he or she still want to hear from me?"

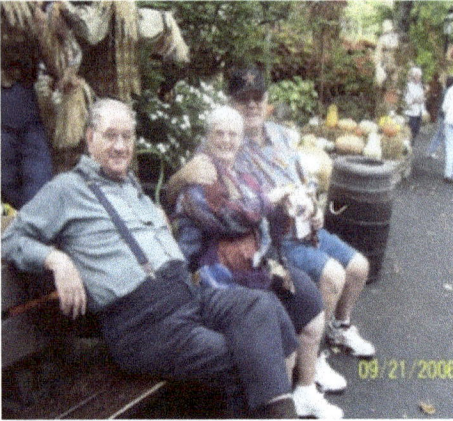

Much has changed as far as my home life. I really enjoyed cooking Russell's favorite dishes: meatloaf, "sketti," and roasts. Now, not so much. For sure, surviving spouses have adjustments to make from day one! It takes time to regroup after our loved one passes; but over time we adjust and feel less like a loose wheel. For me, personally, God has opened new avenues of service. I have more opportunities to speak and share His grace with others. I am writing more and pursuing some hobby interests that have fallen by the wayside.

The bottom line of "My Story" is two-fold:

1. When God brings them to mind, remember to pray for every person you know who has lost a spouse or other loved one.
2. Ask yourself, "What can I do to help them through the adjustment period."

Precious readers, my prayer for you is God's peace in every part of your life. For those of you who have lost loved ones - family and friends alike - I pray for God's comfort and direction in all you do.

Just know there will *always* be one sure thing— GOD'S UNENDING, UNCHANGING LOVE.

Love in the Little Things

"Whoever does not love does not know God,
because God is love." 1 John 4:8 (NIV)

I am very thankful for the parents God gave me. They have passed on to heaven now and I really miss having them around. They raised me and my two sisters to work hard, to be honest and respectful. They were our examples - living the life they taught us to live. They took us to church on Sunday mornings until I was a teenager, then they began to drop us off and pick us up after church services were over. I wasn't sure why they stopped going until years later I found out they were in outs with other church members who had apparently upset them. Did they overreact or did the church member/s step "out of line"? I will never know; but I do know that such situations occur more often than we may realize, with similar results. Where's the LOVE when that happens? Can we forgive in LOVE?

At twelve years of age on Promotion Sunday, Ms. Johnson dismissed our class with prayer. Our heads still bowed, she asked if anyone would like to accept Jesus as their Savior. I raised my hand; and after class was dismissed, she did in fact lead me to the Lord Jesus. I will always be thankful for her LOVING me enough to take me through the steps of salvation.

I have had a normal life of ups and downs that include going to the doctor for stitches, emergency room visits, surgeries and hospital stays. God was with me, always holding my hand in each of those visits right along with my parents, my sisters, my son and daughter or my husband – whoever was available to hold my hand and offer sympathy and communicate my immediate need to the EMTs, nurses and/or doctors. And I felt LOVE. I have gone through a divorce followed by attendance in a divorce counseling group (which I highly recommend) and God LOVED me through it. As hard as it was, those sessions and a year of daily journaling drew me closer to God. He spoke to my heart every day because I was looking to hear from Him. He did not fail me... He LOVED me! After the massive 2011 tornado in Joplin, Missouri, my sisters and I shared caregiving for Dad and Mom for fourteen years. Nine of those years they depended on us totally.

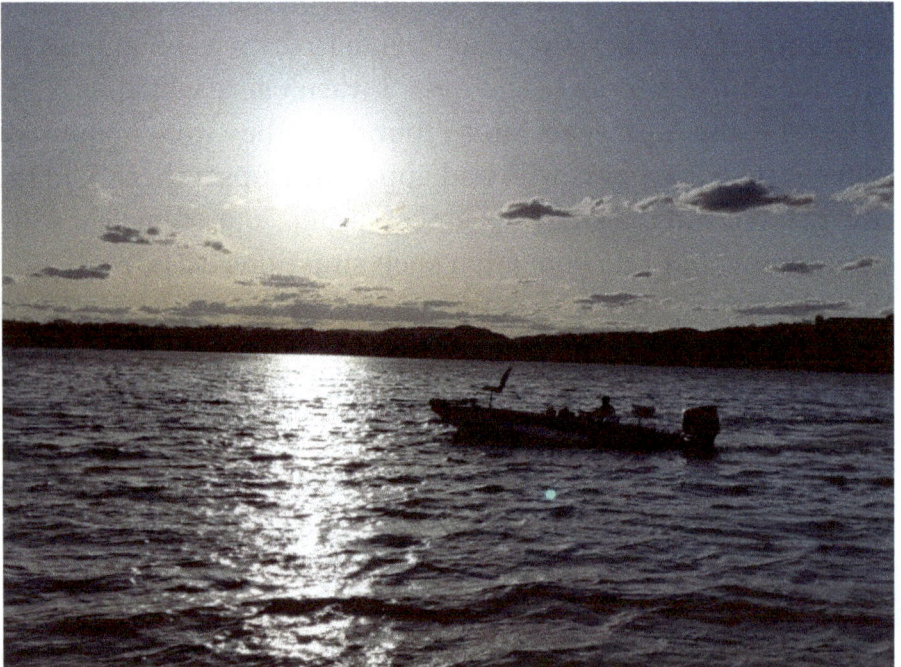

On a much smaller scale, two weeks ago I went on a trip for which my son had loaned me his Suburban SUV – nice! I was a little nervous going on a five-hour trip without much more than a "have a nice trip" and "here are the keys." After the first three hours of the trip, it began to rain – I needed windshield wipers. Quickly I began twisting and turning this and that on the left side of the steering wheel and then on the right. Finally, success! Thankfully I made the trip just fine. Before unpacking the car, I took out the car manual with every intent to educate myself before my return trip. However, on the day I decided to look up a few things, the manual was nowhere to be found. Two weeks later after my return trip – I still had not found what I had done with the manual. I knew well that the Lord saw exactly what I had done with it so, as a last-ditch effort, I begged Him to show me. Do you ever do that?... When all else fails, PRAY? As I am getting older, I find myself concerned with thoughts of losing my "cool" and my "sanity" – so to speak. God did not answer right away; but I did trust that He would soon. I had looked through EVERY piece of luggage and the car more than once, and in my human state of mind there was nowhere else to look. Days later, not forgotten but certainly not on my mind at the time, the Lord practically laid my hand on the manual which was still in the car but between the two front seats. Tears of gratitude instantly streamed down my face. (I am always amazed how much he LOVES me... He LOVES you that way too!) That same day He also brushed my hand over the garage door opener that had been misplaced for longer than the car manual. Again, it took away my breath and LOVE flowed in! God has His reasons for not answering our prayers on the spot or even the next day or two. How much more did I feel His LOVE at those moments than if He had answered right away? I know! Right?

With all the storms we have had in the last couple of months, my eyes have been set on the skies. I have always been in awe of clouds and their formations. As children riding along in the car for an hour or two, my sisters and I would make a game of finding "pictures" in the clouds. The clouds are just one of God's amazing creations, and lately they have been thick, beautiful and even sometimes stormy – I am in awe of God's beauty in nature.

The cumulus and cumulonimbus clouds are so bright and fluffy and sometimes seem to fill the sky - often the sun gives a beautiful, bright light outlining a cloud formation from behind... reminding me that He will one day return in the clouds as He went up into the heavens. How bright the clouds will be then!

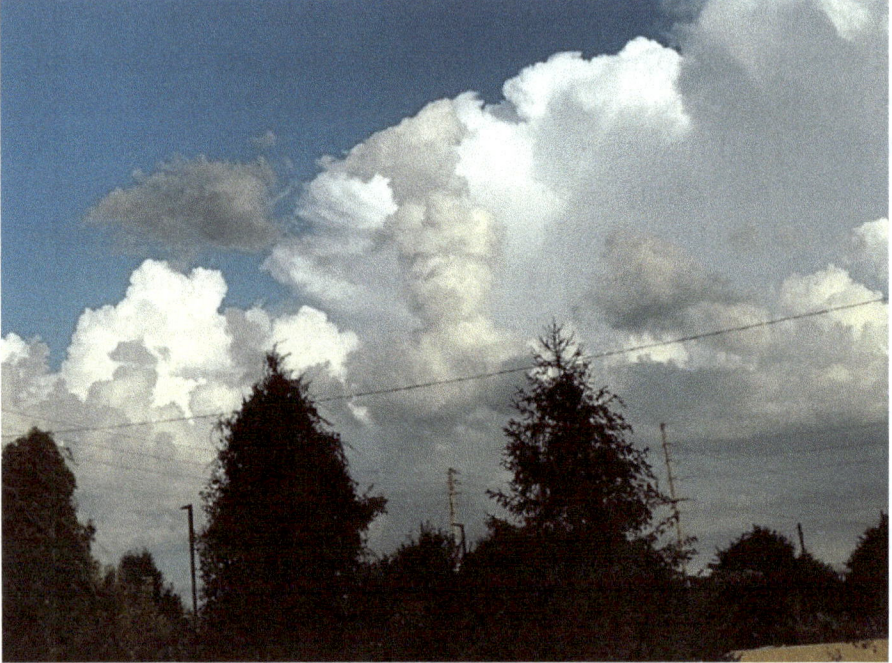

"Look, he is coming with the clouds,' and 'every eye will see him, even those who pierced him;' and all peoples on earth 'will mourn because of him.' So shall it be, Amen." Rev.1:7 NIV

I continually seek ways to stay connected with my adult children, Pam and Scott. Knowing how much I enjoy nature, they have often excitedly shared sunsets, sunrises, rainbows and all sorts of cloud photos, as those pictured as they travel the roadways. They share my feeling of awe when God displays his grandeur for our enjoyment and try to imagine what the majestic show it will be on the day of His return for those who have invited Jesus into their lives.

Of all the great songs of heaven I know, "Awesome God" by Rich Mullins says it so well! When I read the lyrics to this song, I wonder what I will do when I meet God face to face – or what I will say? I wonder... will He say to me "Well Done My Child?"

~Regina Albritton

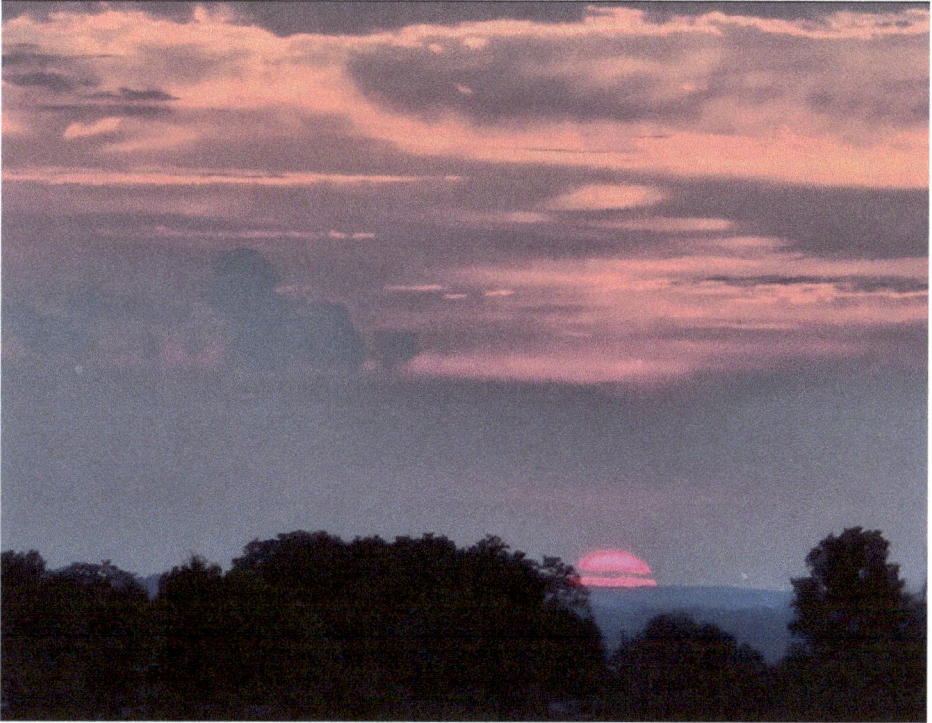

What do you see?

An Encouraging Word

"Commit to the Lord

whatever you do,

and he

will establish your plans."

Proverbs 16:3 (NIV)

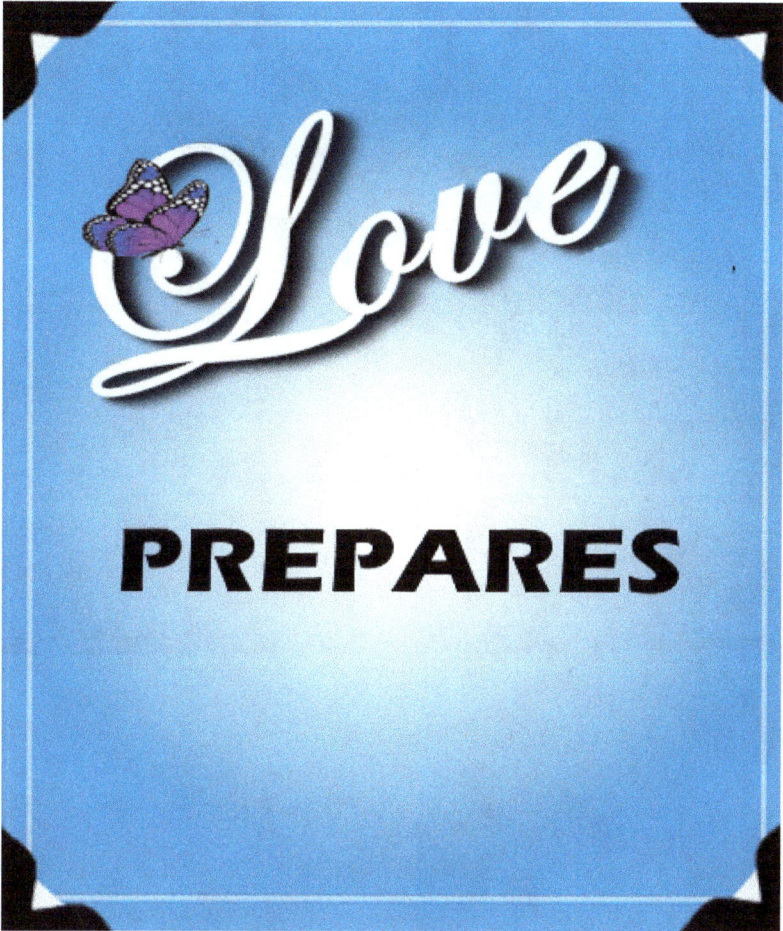

Love

PREPARES

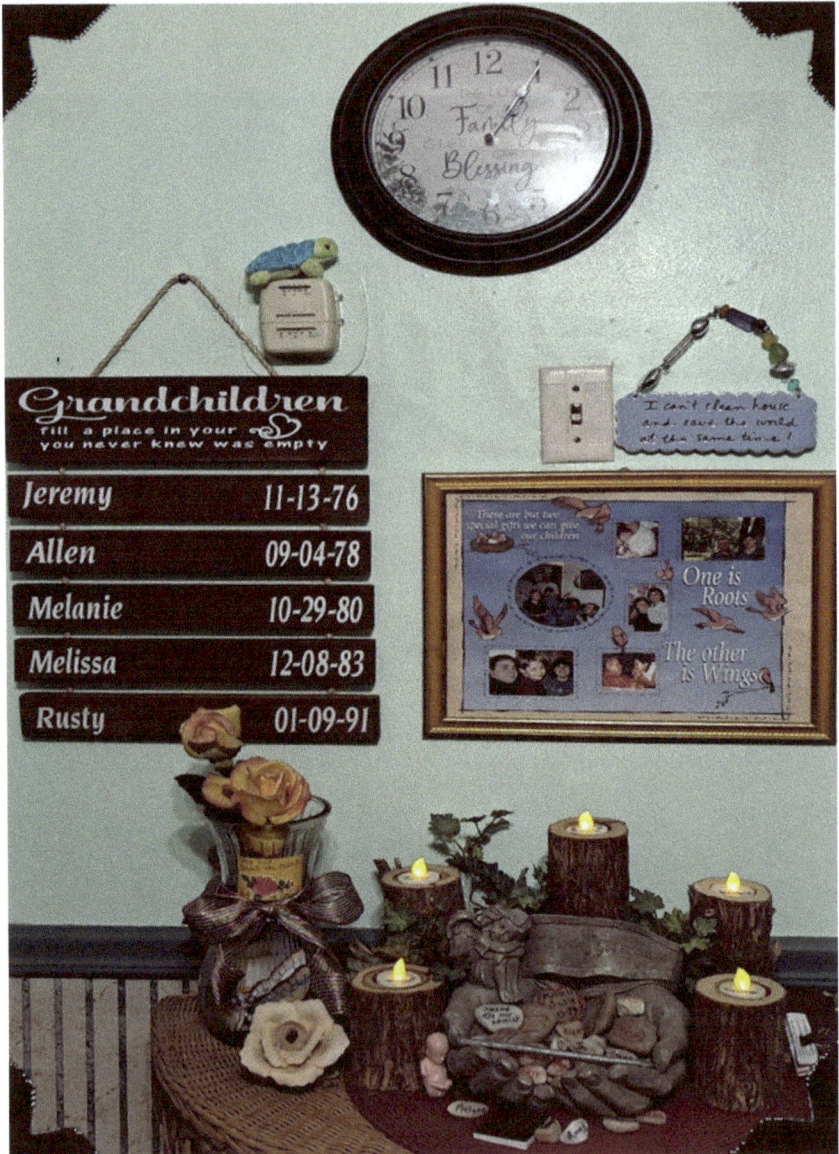

Clock: Family Blessings

Grandchildren
fill a place in your
you never knew was empty

Jeremy	11-13-76
Allen	09-04-78
Melanie	10-29-80
Melissa	12-08-83
Rusty	01-09-91

There are but two special gifts we can give our children

One is Roots

The other is Wings

I can't clean house and save the world at the same time!

It is Wise to Prepare

"There is a time for everything, and a season for every activity under the heavens." Ecclesiastes 3:1 (NIV)

This photo on the left is of my dining room wall. It's the most important wall in my home—my FAMILY! I touch the pebbles with each of their names on them as I head to the kitchen. As I go to bed at night, I light the candles as I pray for each child and their families. My heart's desire is that my family knows Jesus as I do.

But I live alone, far from each of them. I've lived in this community for over twenty-five years. I am well-known and feel loved. However, should something happen to me where I can't communicate, how would my friends know who to contact?

Every day, the unexpected happens to someone. A sudden illness, a vehicle accident, a fire, or a storm. Should full-time care be needed for you, your family, or others, are you ready? Make sure your spouse, family member, or trusted individual has access to your important documents.

Serving over forty years in ministry with my pastor husband, I could tell you horror stories. The most well-intended and seemingly secure families have been blindsided by sudden emergencies. Some have lost homes and possessions because simple issues had been neglected.

May the following pages serve as fuel for thought that produces action. The following pages are intended to stir your thoughts about what is needed in your situation. They are in no way intended to be legal advice. Surround yourself with trustworthy advisers.

Don't miss Wisdom from the Troops; they have been there, and they learned the hard way.

~Susie

Things You Need to Know

"Therefore you also must be ready, for the Son of Man is coming at an hour you do not expect." Matthew 24:44 (NKJV)

Whether you are a spouse or child in the home or live elsewhere and are providing care, there are some essentials that need to be in place. Let this article serve as a reminder to you personally. Each of us needs our own up-to-date information kept in an easily accessible location.

<u>VERY IMPORTANT</u>

1. Set up support for yourself. Caregiving is draining, even if—or maybe especially when—it's for a loved one. Make sure you schedule breaks for yourself. Some nursing homes offer respite care. Call around and see if this helpful benefit is available in your area.
2. Set up expectations with the individual you will be caring for: family member, friend, etc.
3. Discuss times and hours care will be needed.
4. What type of care? Housekeeping, shopping, meal prep, medical care, transportation?
5. Medical authorization: make sure someone can access medical records. Especially if they live across the country from you.
6. Does someone have the Power of Attorney should the patient become unable to make decisions?
7. Is there a Health Care Directive? Do you know where it is? NOTE: Every person needs an Advance Healthcare Directive on file at the hospital or doctor's office.
8. Is there a burial policy? Burial preferences?

9. Are medicines up to date? Who is responsible for giving them? Include prescriptions and Over the Counter (OTC).
    o   Does the person have ANY allergies?
10. Who is to be contacted in an emergency?
    o   Is there a preferred hospital? Physician?

The above are just a few of the questions that need to be addressed when preparing for long-term health care either from a provider or relative. It would be well if every reader of this book would copy this page and make sure his/her family has each of these items in place... That is in a safe place, but easily accessible when needed.

When taking care of Mother, our situation was always revolving. One week she might be totally coherent and could answer any concerns her caregiver might have. Because this was not always the case and I was aware the caregiver may need assistance in the simple tasks, I made cards and posted them in several rooms (bath, bedroom, kitchen). The cards should include a patient's name, address, physician's name, hospital or medical center preferred, medicines, allergies, etc. Vital is current contact information in case of an emergency (doctor, family, or friend who is local.) This is what I posted for Mother. I suggest a similar card on the refrigerator in your purse or vehicle.

Every family and individual should prepare for emergencies. For instance, I live in a community where I am well-known. However, should I need assistance and be incoherent, even my closest friends may not know how to contact my family. I travel all over our county. Should I have a serious accident or pass out, I want someone to be able to help.

Estate Planning

Dr. Neil Franks

The Missouri Baptist Pathway and Dr. Neil Franks granted permission to use the following article: "PREPARING FOR DEATH: A Confident Life."

"Is there anything else I can do for you?"

This simple question people ask us at places like restaurants and stores seems simple and non-confrontational. However, we should consider asking this question more often because someday, it will be the last time we can ask. Described in Luke 16:26 is this reality, "[...] a great chasm has been fixed, in order that those who would pass from here to you may not be able, and none may cross from there to us."

Our whole series in *The Pathway* on the "Confident Life" has focused on growing your confidence in managing money. We cannot leave the topic without discussing what happens when we leave this earth. Now, for most of us, it probably won't be for a while. Almost two-thirds of 70-year-old men and nearly three-fourths of 70-year-old women will live at least another ten years, and more than one-fifth of men will make it to 90.

However, 1% of people under 60 will pass away in the next year around the world, and if estimates are accurate, that represents over three million people, or half the state of Missouri, will pass away. Factor in those over 60, then the number becomes quite large quite quickly, and so do the odds of it being you. That said, as has already been said, the only two things certain in this life are death and taxes. So, if we prepare for taxes, then we need to prepare for death as well.

We call that preparation for death, estate planning.

A good estate plan will have five basic documents. A Will, A Durable Power of Attorney, a Financial Power of Attorney, An Advanced Medical Directive, and a HIPPA authorization. (In addition, many people also benefit from creating a Trust.) Visit www.mbfn.org/legacy to get started today!

If you have already completed all of your documents, you must ensure that all beneficiary designations are accurate and up to date and that family members have access to all the necessary paperwork.

A Confident Financial life starts with FLOW (cash flow, managing your precious dollars). Then, you must make a plan for providing for those you OWE, followed by a plan to GROW those dollars as you SHOW God and others your love through giving generously before you go and spend all eternity with Him.

Wherever you are on your journey, the Missouri Baptist Foundation is here to help you grow in your confidence with all things financial. Give us a call at (573)761-0717 or send us an email at info@mbfn.org to ensure you live a confident life.

~Dr. Neil Franks Baptist Foundation Pathway
    February 19, 2025

Wisdom from the Troops

"Let the one who is wise heed these things and ponder the loving deeds of the LORD." Psalm 107:43 (NIV)

From my readers in their own words.

From *Jacquelyn Lynn* ~

Don't be afraid to bring up hospice, both to your loved one and to the medical team. The doctors in the hospital said it made a big difference to their treatment plan for my dad, knowing that I was ready for hospice to come in. And once hospice is involved, let them do their jobs and help you - they know what they're doing and can/will do things you don't think of that will make the process easier.

This isn't so much advice as just something to be prepared for. I was a caregiver for so many years, and his care needs were escalating, and I got this mindset of "I just have to take care of him until he dies, and then my work is done, and I can relax and rest." Uh, no. He died and then there's all this other stuff you have to do -- the funeral, of course, but more than that. Cleaning out their homes. Disposing of their things. Handling their finances. We were prepared and my father's estate was modest, but there was still SO MUCH to be done, so many calls to make. I spent a lot of time thinking, "I thought I was done, but this is never going to end."

From *Rhonda Hobbs* (Facebook Post) ~

Good morning all my wonderful family and friends!! Today I'm going out to Bodega Bay, saying a prayer and tossing a flower into the sea for Mom. This is her one-year anniversary of going home to be with her Lord and Savior Jesus Christ!! Love you all.

From *Enid Rauh Kelsey* ~

I did think of one thing that helped during Larry's battle with brain cancer. When he would become restless and in pain, I would play Christian music. I could see him relax, which helped give his medicine time to reduce the pain.

From *Karen Dovidio* ~

When my mother was ill, I bought an inexpensive wireless doorbell. I gave her the little push button and placed the speaker near me to hear if she needed help. It was especially needed when I was asleep so I would be awakened by the bell.

From *Linda Buckley* ~

One can use a baby monitor. We used monitors in every room but the bathrooms for our group home of foster teens that were being stepped down through the system.

From *Cindy Medley Ferreri* ~

Real quality bed pads that were soft made life easier when accidents happened. We called them princess pads from *Princess and the Pea*.

From *Cheryl Gardner* ~

PRAYER!! Prayer was the most valued help I received.

Also, very helpful for us was the land line phone that he could use. He could call me on my cell phone when I was out on errands in town.

From *Rebecca Howard* ~

Learn how to check vital signs: blood pressure, oxygen levels, blood sugars. If the person is diabetic, learn how to give insulin shots... etc. Documentation: Make sure and document all care given: medicines, any mental, physical or medical issues that might be going on. Track vital signs, etc.

From *Cathy VanDruff* ~

When you build or buy a home, if possible, consider "aging in that home." This means 4' halls, 3' wide doors, and at least one accessible bathroom or a big enough bathroom to make accessible. That means enough room for a wheelchair and one other person to be together there comfortably.

Keep important documents updated and know where they are. Make sure they can be accessed when needed. TOD (Transfer on Death) on titles is important! If there are assets, know where they are kept. If there is property, know property lines. A relative rented my parent's farmland when Dad quit farming and borrowed his farm equipment, without proper documentation, we could possibly face ownership issues in the future when we try to sell the farm.

From *Jacquelyn Lynn* ~

My father had accounts in one bank and one credit union, and getting the money out -- well, I'll just say I understand why people get violent. He died at the end of March; it is July and I'm STILL waiting for the Treasury Department to send me the money from his savings bonds.

One more piece of advice from a friend of mine whose mother died a couple of years ago -- set up a joint bank account giving you rights of survivorship, so you have access to immediate cash to pay for things. Otherwise, you could have to dip into your own funds and wait for the estate to be settled to get paid back.

From *Susie* -

When taking care of Mother, our situation was always revolving. One day she might be totally coherent and could answer any concerns her caregiver might have; the next she was blank. I made cards and posted them in several rooms (bath, bedroom, kitchen). The cards had patient's name, address, physician's name, hospital or medical center preferred, medicines, allergies, etc. Current contact information (doctor, family, or friend) is vital in case of an emergency.

An Encouraging Word

"We

LOVE

Because

HE

first loved

us."

I John 4:19 (NIV)

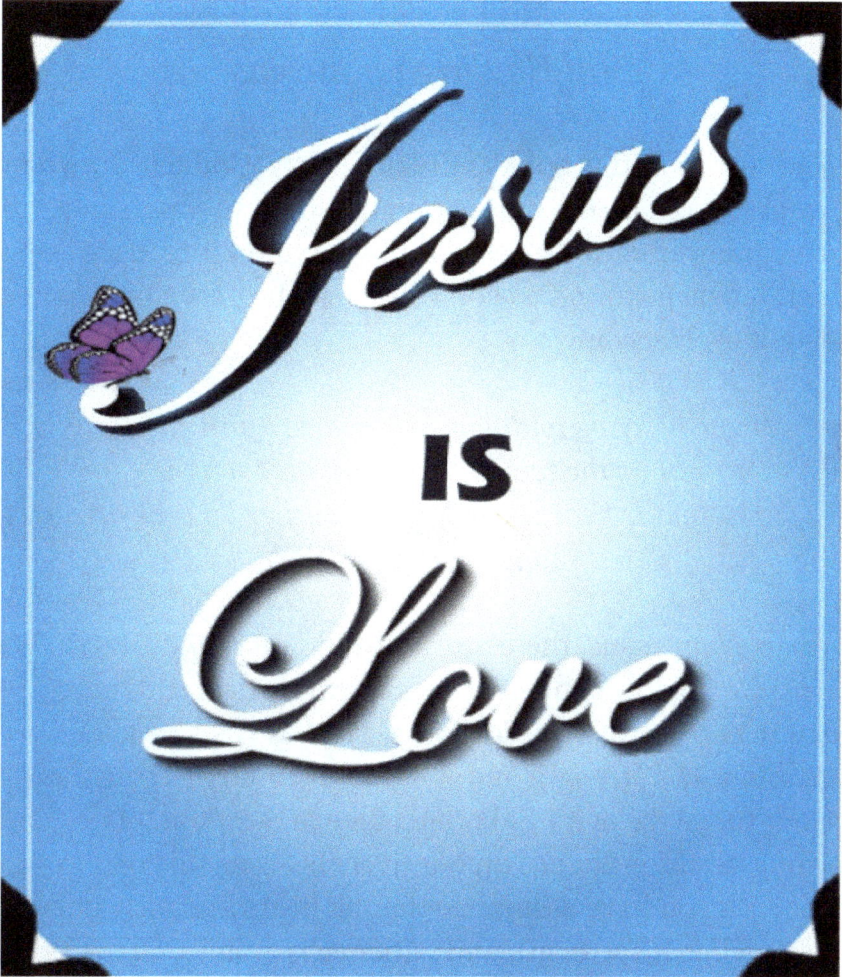

Jesus Loves You

"Greater love hath no man than this, that a man lay down his life for his friends." John 15:13 (KJV)

And He did that for you.

The stories in this book are real. Clearly, God has drawn men and women from across our country to share very personal, often heartbreaking situations. Jesus is the common thread we see throughout each story. Did you recognize the peace that comes at the end of each account?

"Peace I leave with you, My peace I give to you;
not as the world gives do I give to you.
Let not your heart be troubled, neither let it be afraid."
John 14:27 (NKJV)

Apart from Jesus, these stories would be very different. We do not have it within ourselves to show the grace and mercy needed to care for others like Jesus. It takes His love and compassion, His strength and wisdom. I would be remiss as I close out this writing if I did not challenge our thoughts regarding Jesus' influence on our lives. Is Jesus this real to you and me? Do you have assurance that he hears and answers your groaning when all strength and patience is gone? Consider the truths found in John 15:11-17 ASV. Pray with me through each verse. Make it personal.

"These things have I spoken to you, that My joy may remain in you, and that your joy may be full.

This is My commandment, that you love one another as I have loved you.

Greater love has no one than this, than to lay down one's life for his friends.

You are My friends if you do whatever I command you.

No longer do I call you servants, for a servant does not know what his master is doing; but I have called you friends, for all things that I heard from My Father I have made known to you.

You did not choose Me, but I chose you and appointed you that you should go and bear fruit, and that your fruit should remain, that whatever you ask the Father in My name He may give you.

These things I command you, that you love one another."

John 15:11-17 (NKJV)

May you seek God's wisdom in your every decision, however small it may seem. May God's Spirit touch your heart through these stories and draw you and your family closer to him. May you truly accept His boundless love as found through His only son, Jesus Christ.

Jesus loves YOU more than words can say. His love is pure, undefiled, and freely given. He is waiting for you to accept it.

~Susie

Let me hear from you.

susie@susiekinslowadams.com

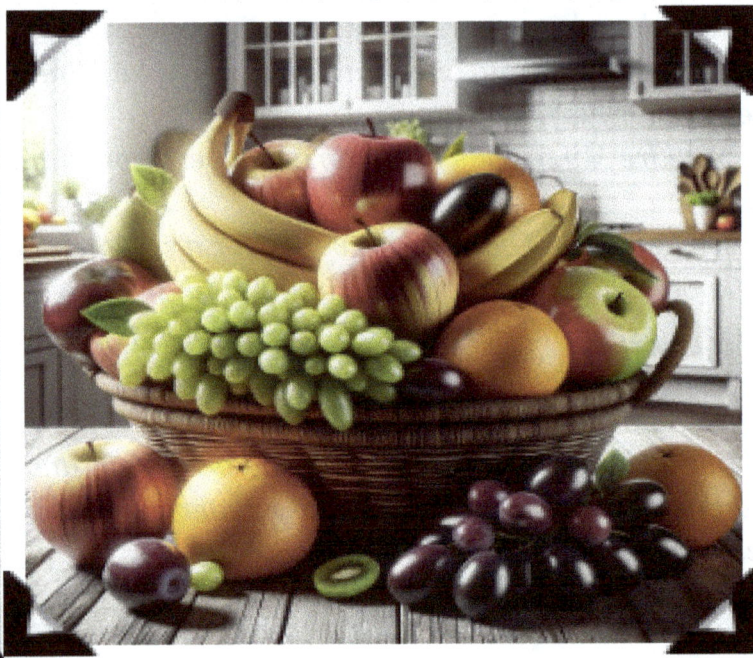

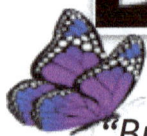

"But the **fruit of the Spirit** is love, joy, peace, longsuffering, gentleness, goodness, faith, Meekness, temperance: against such there is no law."

Galatians 5:22-23 (KJV)

RESOURCES

Where to Find Helpful Resources

Where no counsel is, the people fall: but in the multitude of counselors there is safety." Proverbs 11:14 (KJV)

This short list of resources is by no means conclusive. Each contact you make concerning you or your loved one's health needs to be bathed in prayer. Have good counsel around to help you choose wisely. Often, what's needed will simply be someone to encourage you.

LOCAL CHURCH AND MINISTERIAL ALLIANCES: Knowing what is available in your immediate community is key. Become aware of the help available in your area.

THE DEPARTMENT OF HEALTH AND SOCIAL SERVICES, DIVISION OF AGING, DEPARTMENT OF HUMAN RESOURCES, SENIOR CITIZENS' SERVICE ORGANIZATIONS may offer programs not listed separately..

LOCAL PHONE DIRECTORY: Look for listings under Health Care Facilities, Home Health Services, Hospital Equipment and Supplies-Retail.

CAREGIVER.ORG For more than 40 years, FCA (Family Caregiver Alliance) has provided services to family caregivers of adults with physical and cognitive impairments, such as Parkinson's, stroke, Alzheimer's, and other types of dementia. Their services include assessment, care planning, direct care skills, wellness programs, respite services, and legal/financial consultation vouchers. FCA is a longtime advocate for caregivers in the areas of policy, health and social system development, research, and public awareness, on the state, national, and international levels.

FREEDOMCARE.COM is an excellent site to determine whether you or a family member will qualify as a paid caregiver for your loved one. The FreedomCare program is for those on Medicaid.

HEALTHINAGING.ORG is a trusted source for up-to-date information and advice on health and aging, created by the American Geriatrics Society's Health in Aging Foundation. This foundation features educational materials for older adults and caregivers, as well as information on finding a geriatric healthcare professional in your area. These tools have been reviewed by geriatrics healthcare professionals and members of the American Geriatrics Society (AGS)—a community of experts in the care we all need as we age.

HOSPICEFOUNDATION.ORG is an informative link to help you understand the many facets of hospice care.

HOPE4WIDOWS.COM - A Place For Widows To Find Community - WINGS book (Widows In New Growth Seasons)

SENIORSBLUEBOOK.COM - Since 1983, the Seniors Blue Book has helped Millions of Seniors & Caregivers navigate the confusing world of Senior Housing, Senior Care, Resources, and Services. Let them be your guide in helping you find the information you need when you need it most.

UNITEDWAY.COM and AARP have joined together to sponsor 211. Check their website for details.

CALENDAR/DAY CLOCKS – There is a large variety of clocks available that prominently display the month, day, date, and time.

REMINDER CLOCKS can also show medicine times and other helpful information.

Thank You!

Thank you for reading *What Love Looks Like*. I hope you were blessed, encouraged, or inspired to share it with someone else! I would be delighted if you could write a kind review.

If you enjoyed these true stories, you may also enjoy my other books.

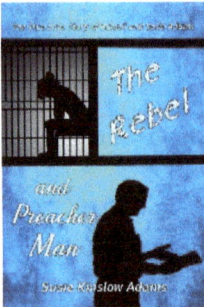

The Rebel and Preacher Man:

The True Love Story of Russell & Susie Adams

How can a rebellious young woman in her thirties meet a godly preacher man in his fifties and fall in love? How can an unchurched girl become the preacher's wife in only a few months? Only when God orchestrates the whole plan. An amazing true story of love and resilience, and how the Lord works in amazing ways!

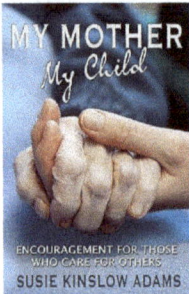

My Mother, My Child is an easy-to-read, very personal book that will help and encourage you, whether you are an adult caring for aging parents, *a* parent of small children, a professional caregiver, or an individual wanting to help others.

The thought-provoking questions and insights at the end of each chapter are suitable for individual or group study. Every person is entitled to adequate care and respect regardless of age or circumstance. *My Mother, My Child* is written from the perspective of the author as she learns to be the caregiver to her aging mother suffering from Alzheimer's Disease.

Available on Amazon or Barnes and Noble in print or digital.

Meet the Author

Award-winning Author of *My Mother My Child, The Rebel and Preacher Man,* and two children's scripture activity books.

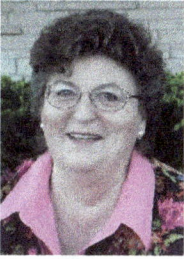

Susie Kinslow Adams is a gifted and award-winning author, writer, speaker, and storyteller. She worked alongside her husband, Dr. Russell Adams, as he pastored churches and served as Director of Missions for the Dallas County Association of Southern Baptists. Susie led women's Bible studies and directed women's retreats in California, Oklahoma, and Missouri.

As an active member of the Springfield Writers' Guild and American Christian Writers, Susie has won numerous writing contests. Her books: *My Mother, My Child* (a practical guide and workbook on dealing with Alzheimer's), *The Rebel and Preacher Man: The True Love Story of Russell and Susie Adams,* and two children's activity books, *Patches' Joyland Express,* and *Patches' Farmland Adventures,* are available on Amazon. Another children's activity book is planned for release in the future.

COMING:

What FAITH Looks Like

Do you have a story that must be told? I look forward to reading it. It might be selected for the next anthology!

Send stories any time:
susie@susiekinslowadams.com or mail to
Susie K. Adams, P.O. Box 138, Buffalo, MO 65622

CHILDREN'S BOOKS BY SUSIE

Look for these wonderful books on Amazon.

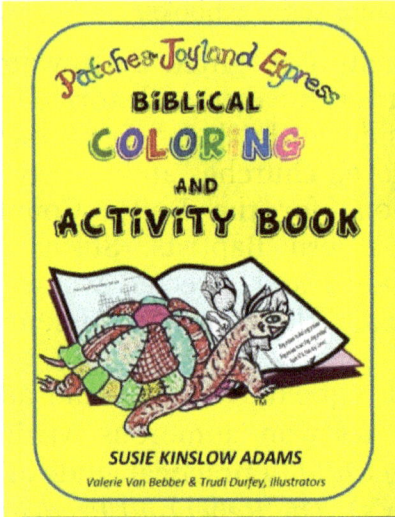

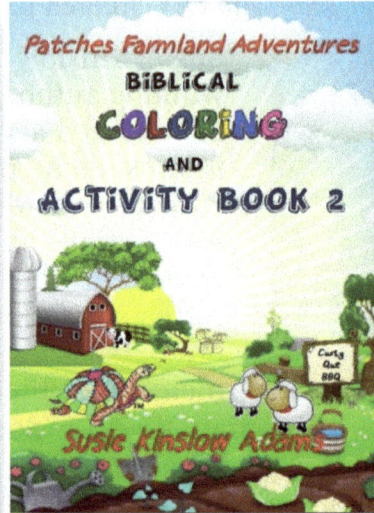

Patches, the turtle, has designed
biblical coloring and activity books for children of all ages and the
young at heart! Filled with coloring pages, puzzles, and inspiring
stories, he wants families to have fun together.

COMING: *PATCHES FRIENDSHIP* – Patches' best friend is
Pockets, the kangaroo. Get ready for more fun as they discover new
friends!

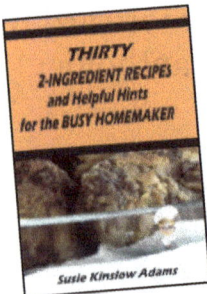

More information and informative
articles are available at
www.susiekinslowadams.com.

Sign up for her encouraging blog and
receive a free cookbook.

www.ingramcontent.com/pod-product-compliance
Lightning Source LLC
Chambersburg PA
CBHW060607200326
41521CB00007B/681